COVID-19

THE PANDEMIC

For information about permission to reproduce sections
from this book, email abhagatmd@gmail.com.
Thank you for your support of the author's rights.

Book design by Ivica Jandrijevic

ISBN 978-1-64059-023-6 (paperback)
ISBN 978-1-64059-024-3 (e-book)

COVID-19
THE PANDEMIC

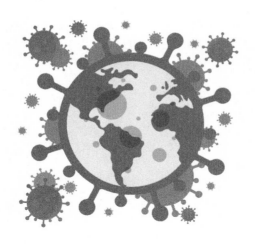

ITS IMPACT ON HEALTH,
ECONOMY, AND THE WORLD

ABHISHEK BHAGAT, M.D.

For humanity: a snapshot of COVID-19 and its impact in 2020. May we learn from this pandemic and collectively prevent future threats to the pale blue dot we call home.

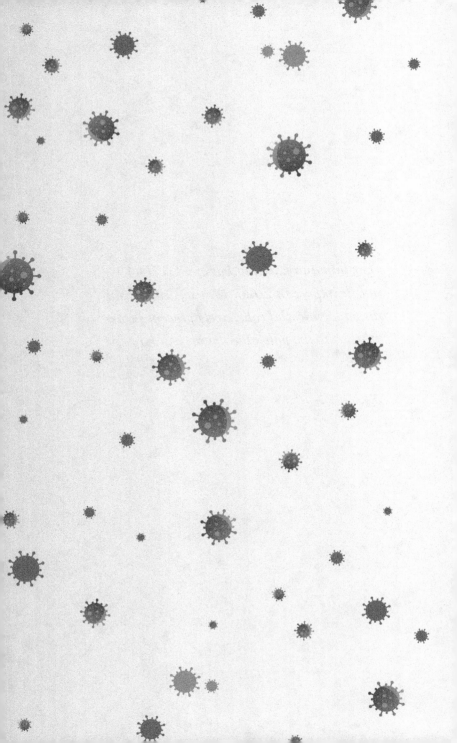

CONTENTS

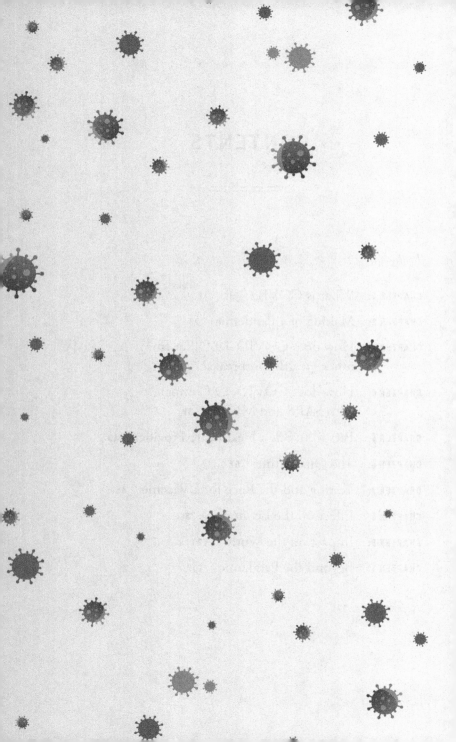

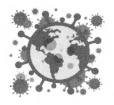

PREFACE

I N LIGHT OF the ongoing pandemic that is affecting billions of people worldwide, my goal for writing this book was to create awareness. Maybe it's just the physician in me, but when this pandemic first started, I was filled with questions such as why and how? I'm sure COVID-19 has, in some shape or form, impacted you or one of your loved ones. Maybe your uncle became infected with the virus, or your best friend lost her job, or perhaps you could not attend that concert you were excited about. It has touched all of us. Here, you will find a distillation of the pertinent information about this outbreak that we have learned until now. What exactly is COVID-19? How did it all begin? How was this so much worse than our other recent outbreaks? When are we getting a vaccine? What lessons can we learn from this? Will something like this happen again? I have done my best to make this information easy to digest in short bite-sized chapters. My goal is to inform and to educate, not to profit when millions have lost their jobs. All of the proceeds from the sale of these books will be donated to charity. Let's prevent future catastrophes. Let's make the world a better place.

WHAT IS COVID-19?

This is not the end. It is not even the beginning of the end. But it is, perhaps, the end of the beginning.

Winston Churchill

COVID-19 IS AN acronym for **co**rona**vi**rus **d**isease, and 19 is short for 20**19**, the year it was discovered. SARS-CoV-2 (**s**evere **a**cute **r**espiratory **s**yndrome **c**orona**vi**rus **2**), also known as the 2019 novel coronavirus, is the virus responsible for this disease. Why does the virus have a different name than the disease? Viruses generally have different names than the diseases they cause. For example, varicella zoster is a virus that causes shingles. Viruses are named based on their genetic structure to ease the development of diagnostic tests and vaccines. Diseases are named in order to facilitate discussion about disease prevention and treatment.[1]

SARS-CoV-2 is a newly discovered member of the *Coronaviridae* family, which includes six previously known human-infecting viruses. Four of the previously known human-infecting coronaviruses typically result in common cold symptoms such as sneezing, runny nose, and nasal congestion. The more harmful strains are SARS-CoV-1 (resulting in the 2002 SARS epidemic), MERS-CoV (resulting in the Middle Eastern Respiratory Syndrome outbreak), and the newly discovered SARS-CoV-2.

Coronaviruses have crown-like projections on their surfaces, deriving the word *corona*, Latin for crown. COVID-19 is a zoonotic disease, i.e., a disease that can be transferred from other animals to humans. SARS-CoV-2 shares 80% similar DNA with SARS-CoV-1, also, 96% genetic similarity with the bat coronavirus (Bat-CoV RaTG13), and 91% similarity with a coronavirus detected in anteater-like animals called pangolins (Pangolin-CoV).[2,3] Similar to SARS-CoV-1 and MERS-CoV, the available data suggests that bats appear to be the likely reservoir for SARS-CoV-2. However, it is unlikely the bats directly transmitted the virus to humans. It is believed that bats carried the virus to another animal, an intermediate host, which subsequently infected humans. It is believed that SARS-CoV-1 jumped from bats to Malayan pangolins and then underwent genetic mixing (recombination) before infecting humans.[4]

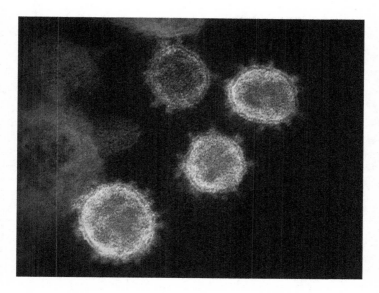

*Transmission electron microscope image of SARS-CoV-2
virus particles isolated from a patient. Credit: NIAID*

Is COVID-19 truly so much worse than the original
SARS outbreak? In the initial phases of the COVID-19
pandemic, public health officials utilized similar interventions used to manage the SARS outbreak.[5] However, despite the application of similar interventions to control the
spread of the disease, the trajectories of the two outbreaks
diverged considerably. After 8,400 cases and 916 deaths
worldwide, the US Centers for Disease Control and Prevention (CDC) considered the SARS epidemic contained
four months after issuing global alerts. In contrast, within
three months of being declared a public health emergency,
there were more than three million cases and more than
200,000 deaths due to COVID-19.

HOW DID THE VIRUS SPREAD SO QUICKLY?

There are several explanations behind the profound transmission of the novel coronavirus. First, along with being the largest city in Central China, Wuhan is a major transportation hub. It is home to one of the largest airports and railway stations in the region. China's high-speed rail system extends more than 10 times the distance in 2020 than it did in 2003. In 2003, the combined length of highways in China was 30,000 kilometers, while in 2020, it's more than 140,000 kilometers. In 2003, China had seven million international passengers. In 2020, it has more than 63 million.[6] Given these circumstances, today the virus is able to travel much quicker and farther, along with its human host. Being a large metropolitan city, Wuhan incorporates concentrated living and working conditions – expediting transmission of the virus. These factors, along with massive gatherings just prior to the lockdown, further exacerbated the spread.[7]

Another critical reason why COVID-19 has spread so vastly is the asymptomatic transmission, which is transmission of the virus from a person who had not developed symptoms. No SARS cases have been reported to be contagious before the patient developed symptoms. In contrast, SARS-CoV-2 has shown to be transmittable before the onset of symptoms. Because of this, isolation when the person is showing the symptoms may be too late to contain the spread.

Reaching more than 200 countries within three months, COVID-19 advanced at unprecedented speed.

Various studies suggest that air traffic played an essential role in the spread of the virus. Stronger connections with China were associated with earlier dates of pandemic spread.[8] Thailand and Japan were the most frequent flight destinations from Wuhan, in addition to being two of the earliest countries to start showing infections outside of China. As the world continues to further globalize, viruses will travel with just as much speed as passengers across the globe.

On average, each infected person transmits the virus to three additional individuals. In epidemiological terms, the mean basic reproduction number (R_0) is 3.28.[9] But the contagiousness of the virus will vary based on factors such as the population's density, contact frequency, etc. It will be more contagious in dense cities compared to remote villages. R_0 (pronounced "R-naught") is the average number of new infections from a single infected person. An R_0 value less than one indicates that the outbreak is shrinking since each infected person is infecting less than one person.[10] Whereas an R_0 above one indicates that the outbreak is expanding – each person is infecting more than one person.

The time between becoming infected with this novel virus and then showing symptoms (incubation period) is, on average, five-to-six days. However, some people may take up to 14 days to show symptoms, and a few may not show symptoms at all![11] If some people have the virus but do not show signs and are, therefore, not quarantined, they can contribute to further spread. Because of this, the asymptomatic or pre-symptomatic transmission of the virus is particularly concerning.

Which virus is more lethal to humanity - a virus that kills its host the same day of infection or a virus that does not even begin to show symptoms until a week after infecting before sickening and killing its host? If you don't show symptoms for a week, the virus has a seven-day period to covertly infect numerous others. Generally speaking, viruses need host cells to survive and replicate. Therefore, it's in the virus' best interest to not kill its host – allowing its own survival and to not sicken its host (at least not immediately) – allowing for occult transmission.

How does the virus spread? Human-to-human transmission of SARS-CoV-2 is generally through respiratory droplets and fomites (contaminated objects such as doorknobs, clothing, etc.). Transmission through respiratory droplets occurs with close contact (within one meter) with an infected person who has respiratory symptoms (such as coughing or sneezing) or is talking. Airborne transmission through aerosols (smaller-sized droplets) means germ particles remain in the air for more extended periods and spread farther. At this point, it is not yet clear whether the virus can be transmitted through aerosols or not. However, it does have aerosol distribution and may possibly reach a distance of up to four meters (13 feet).[12] Infection from blood, urine, and stool particles is also possible. We touch our faces hundreds of times a day. This allows for the virus to be easily transmitted through fomites. SARS-CoV-2's stability has been studied in different environmental conditions. The virus was demonstrated to remain viable in aerosols for at least three hours. It was also found to be more stable on plastic and stainless steel than on copper or cardboard surfaces – detected for up to 72 hours on plastic (although the quantity of the virus had markedly diminished). No viable virus was detected on copper after four hours.[13]

WHAT ARE THE SYMPTOMS OF COVID-19?

The most common symptoms seen with this infection are fever (seen in 83% of patients), cough (60%), and fatigue (38%). Other symptoms, seen in less than 30% of cases, are increased phlegm (sputum) production, shortness of breath, and muscle aches (myalgia). No symptoms were seen in 5.6% of patients. Commonly reported abnormalities seen in blood tests are reduced immune cell (lymphocyte) count and elevated inflammatory (C-reactive protein) and tissue injury (lactate dehydrogenase) markers.

The most common findings on chest computed tomography (CT) scans were areas of haziness (ground-glass opacities) in the lungs and pneumonia.[14] Fluid build-up in the tiny air sacs (alveoli) of lungs preventing adequate oxygen from reaching the blood (acute respiratory distress syndrome [ARDS]) has been reported as the most common significant complication. Additionally, data from China suggests that 3.6% of cases resulted in death. The case fatality rate (CFR) is the proportion of deaths due to a disease. In the US, 1.8% to 3.4% of infections have led to death.[15] Keep in mind that the percentage of severe cases, complications, and deaths change if the patient population in focus changes. For example, if you only

COVID-19 Symptoms

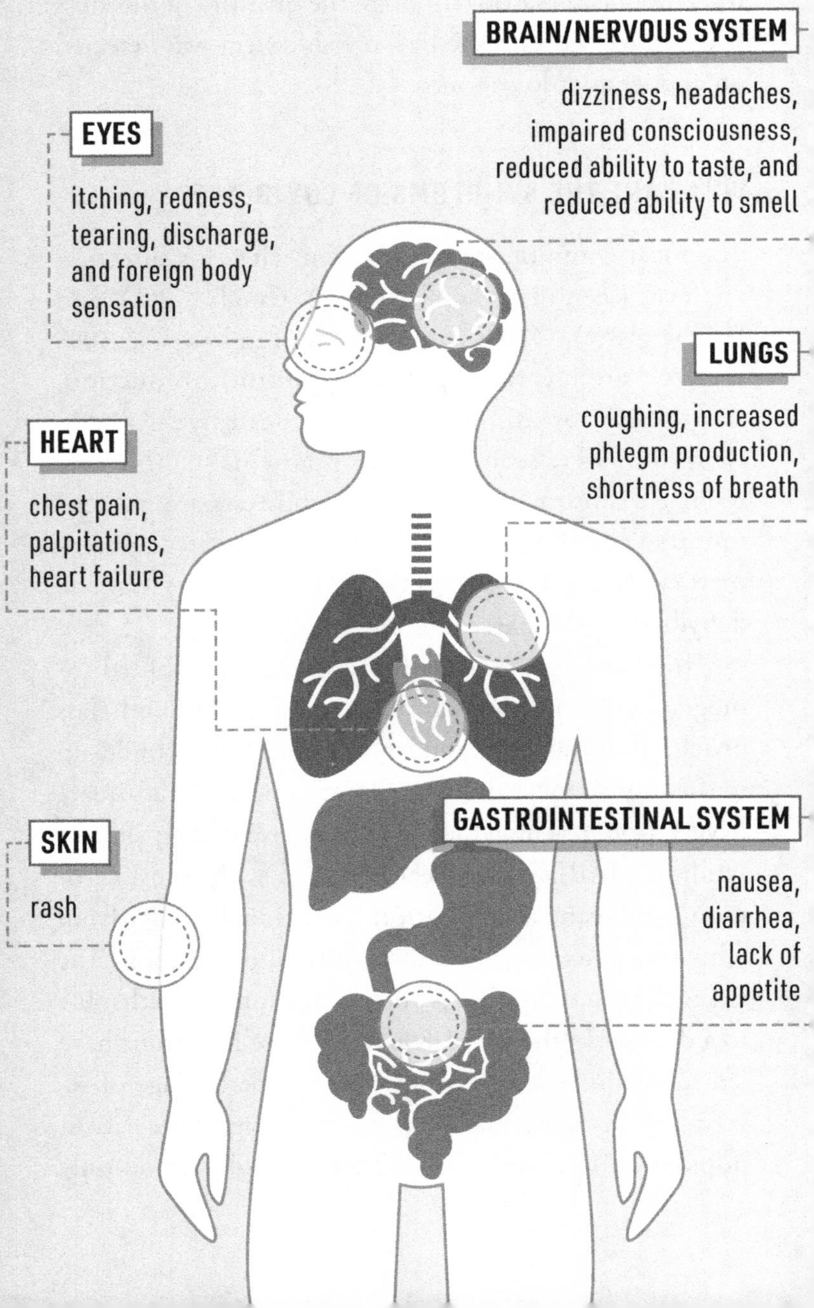

BRAIN/NERVOUS SYSTEM

dizziness, headaches, impaired consciousness, reduced ability to taste, and reduced ability to smell

EYES

itching, redness, tearing, discharge, and foreign body sensation

LUNGS

coughing, increased phlegm production, shortness of breath

HEART

chest pain, palpitations, heart failure

GASTROINTESTINAL SYSTEM

nausea, diarrhea, lack of appetite

SKIN

rash

look at the elderly infected population, the severe case and death proportions will be markedly higher.

The novel coronavirus also appears to disproportionately impact people with prior health conditions. Individuals with underlying high blood pressure (hypertension), diabetes, heart disease (for example, a history of heart attack), lung disease (chronic obstructive pulmonary disease [COPD]), and cerebrovascular disease (for example, a history of stroke) appear to be at an increased risk not only for catching the virus but also for having severe disease compared to their healthier counterparts.[16,17]

Brain/nervous system: Affected in 36% of hospitalized patients and more commonly in severe cases. The most common symptoms in order of frequency: dizziness, headaches, impaired consciousness, reduced ability to taste (hypogeusia), reduced ability to smell (hyposmia), and rarely, strokes or seizures.[18]

Eyes: Affected in about 7% of patients. Symptoms include itching (63%), redness (38%), tearing (38%), discharge (25%), and a *something in my eye* (foreign body) sensation (25%).[19]

Heart: Patients may present with chest pain (15%) and palpitations.[20] COVID-19 inflicts injury to the heart muscle in about 8% of hospitalized patients.[21] Also, 17% of patients developed abnormal heart rhythms.[22] The weakening of the heart's pumping ability (heart failure) has also been reported in 23% of hospitalized patients.[23] The actual number of heart attacks has not been clearly reported but appears to be low.[24] Very rarely, abrupt stopping of the heart function (cardiac arrest) has also been reported.

Lungs: The main target of COVID-19. Coughing is one of the most common symptoms (60% of patients). Increased phlegm production is seen in 27% of patients, and shortness of breath is seen in 25%. A runny nose is seen in 4% of patients. Coughing up blood and nasal congestion have been reported as occurring rarely (2%). A life-threatening complication in which fluid builds up within the air sacs in the lungs preventing enough oxygen from reaching the blood (ARDS) is the most common complication seen in almost 16% of the patients.[25]

Gastrointestinal system: Affected in about 40% of patients. The reported symptoms in order of frequency are nausea, diarrhea, lack of appetite, abdominal pain, belching, and vomiting.[26]

Skin: Affected in about 20% of patients.[27] Small, reddish, and flat or slightly-raised circular spots (morbilliform rash) is the most common skin finding seen in 36% of patients presenting with skin manifestations. Other kinds of rashes, such as small blisters (35%) or hives (10%), have also been reported. Net-like reddish-blue skin discoloration has also been rarely reported (3%). Most of these rashes occurred on the trunk (69%)

while others occurred on hands and feet (19%). In patients who did develop skin manifestations, for 69% of them, the skin changes occurred after the respiratory symptoms.[28]

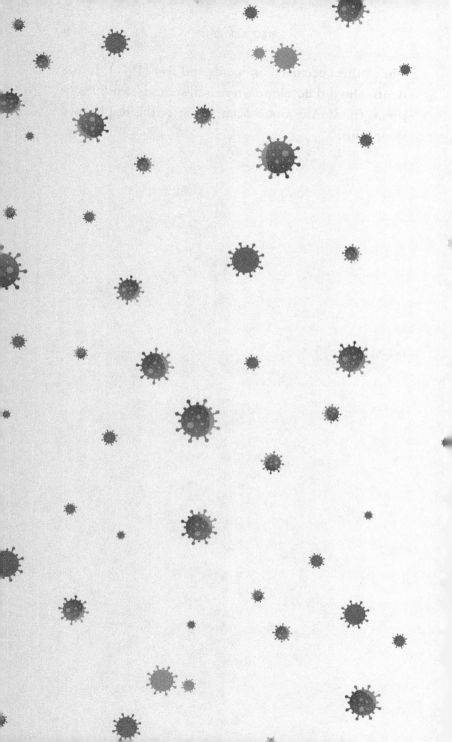

MAKING OF A PANDEMIC

The worst pandemic in modern
history was the Spanish Flu of 1918,
which killed tens of millions of people.
Today, with how interconnected the
world is, it would spread faster.

Bill Gates

THE SPRING FESTIVAL on January 25th became an un-forgettable memory to Chinese citizens as they were urged by their government to stay indoors for many weeks, and public transportation was shut down due to increasing numbers of infections and deaths from a new coronavirus. What started as a viral outbreak in Wuhan, China, rapidly disseminated as a pandemic to more than

200 countries. A similar pattern of a mysterious pneumonia-like illness originating from a wet market in China and quickly spreading to other countries had been observed from 2002 to 2003. That was SARS.

In late December 2019, increasing numbers of pneumonia cases due to unknown etiology emerged in Wuhan, Hubei, China. Several patients had been linked to the Huanan Seafood Wholesale Market. "Wet markets," such as this one, tend to be very condensed and crowded, usually selling both dead and live animals – pigs, chickens, dogs, and fresh seafood, among others. Few of the markets slaughter the animals on site. Some wet markets, including the Huanan Market, also sold wild animals such as snakes, beavers, civets, and baby crocodiles. Live and dead animals mixing with humans in a crowded setting with questionable sanitary practices is a perfect nidus for zoonotic diseases to emerge.

On January 1, 2020, Huanan Market was shut down due to concerns for the market being the source of the outbreak. On January 7, 2020, after ruling out other germs such as influenza, SARS-CoV-1, and MERS-CoV, the Chinese identified the culprit behind these new cases as novel coronavirus. The number of people who were catching the virus and were dying from the disease started escalating, particularly in the Hubei province. Additionally, viral cases started emerging in other Asian countries, including Thailand, South Korea, and Japan. Wuhan is one of China's ten most inhabited cities, with a population of 11 million people. For comparison, New York City's population is 8.3 million, and

London's population is nine million. On January 23rd, Wuhan was closed off by the Chinese authorities. Air travel, trains, buses, subways, and ferries were all suspended. Mandatory closures of public venues, such as restaurants, cinemas, bookstores, and schools, were implemented. Additional attempts to further contain the virus included lockdown and suspension of public transportation in two nearby cities: Huanggang (population of 6.3 million) and Ezhou (population of 1.1 million).[29] Limiting movement through measures, such as travel restrictions, reduced public transport, and curfews were then extended to additional provinces, in total affecting more than 50 million Chinese. In effect, the world witnessed the largest quarantine known to mankind.

Quarantine, from the Italian *quaranta*, meaning 40, of the ill is not a new practice and has been used in some shape or form since at least The Middle Ages. During the bubonic plague of the 14th century, ships arriving in Venice from infected ports were required to sit at anchor for 40 days before passengers were allowed to disembark. A plague hospital (lazaretto) first emerged on Croatia's coast, and the idea was soon adopted in other nearby regions. During the cholera outbreaks of the 18th century, travelers who had contact with infected people or who had arrived from cholera endemic areas were forced into lazarettos. During the 20th century, the Spanish Flu (H1N1 influenza) resulted in many measures similar to what we're using today, including school and church closures, public gatherings being brought to a halt, and the use of physical (social) distancing. However, due to the measures being uncoordinated and implemented too late, infections due to influenza were rampant.[30]

On January 30, 2020, the WHO affirmed the new coronavirus outbreak as a public health emergency of international concern. This made the novel coronavirus the fifth public health emergency declared within the past decade, joining the outbreaks of Ebola in West Africa (2014), polio (2014), Zika (2016), and the re-emergence of Ebola from the Democratic Republic of Congo (2019).

The toll this pandemic is taking is not similar for all socioeconomic groups; it appears to be greater on lower socioeconomic segments. In the US, these groups mostly consist of blacks, Hispanics, and Native Americans.[31] Generally speaking, lower socioeconomic groups tend to consume poorer diets, exercise less, smoke more, and have more psychological stress.[32] Additionally, low-income individuals are also more likely to have more than one physical or mental health condition 10-15 years earlier than people residing in more affluent areas.[33] Therefore, it is understandable why individuals from lower socioeconomic groups would be more susceptible to the viral illness.

How long will the pandemic last? At this point, it's difficult to say, but do not be surprised by an 18-to-24 month timeline.[34] The duration and peaks of the pandemic will be influenced by mitigation strategies varying across the globe, the timing of a widely available and effective vaccine, and the availability of testing. Additionally, the knowledge of whether an infected person develops immunity (and if so, for how long) will also affect the pandemic timeline.

POTENTIAL COVID-19 RESURGENCE SCENARIOS:

Scenario 1: Following the first wave of COVID-19 in the Spring of 2020, similar repetitive waves will follow over a one-to-two-year period. The height of the wave (indicating the number of infections) will influence the reinforcement or loosening of periodic lockdowns and mitigation measures.

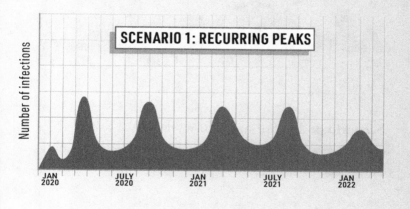

Scenario 2: After the wave seen in the Spring of 2020, when non-pharmaceutical interventions (NPIs), such as physical distancing and travel restrictions are eased, a larger wave of COVID-19 infections in the fall or winter will follow. The larger wave will then be followed by additional smaller waves. The larger wave will necessitate reinstating lockdowns and other mitigation strategies. A similar pattern was observed with the Spanish Flu in 1918 – 1919. Most of the US deaths during the 1918 pandemic

occurred due to the second wave.[35] The Asian Flu and the
Swine Flu pandemics followed a similar pattern.

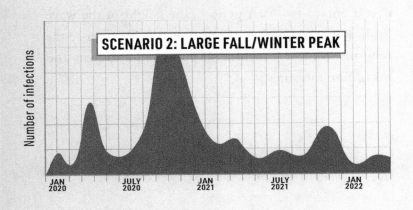

Scenario 3: The Spring 2020 wave will be followed by
miniature waves indicating a smaller number of ongoing
outbreaks.[36]

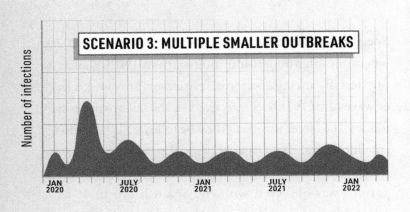

A UK study funded by the Bill & Melinda Gates Foundation found that if NPIs in China had been implemented one, two, or three weeks earlier, cases could have been reduced by 66%, 86%, and 95%, respectively. This would have considerably limited the geographical spread of the virus.[37]

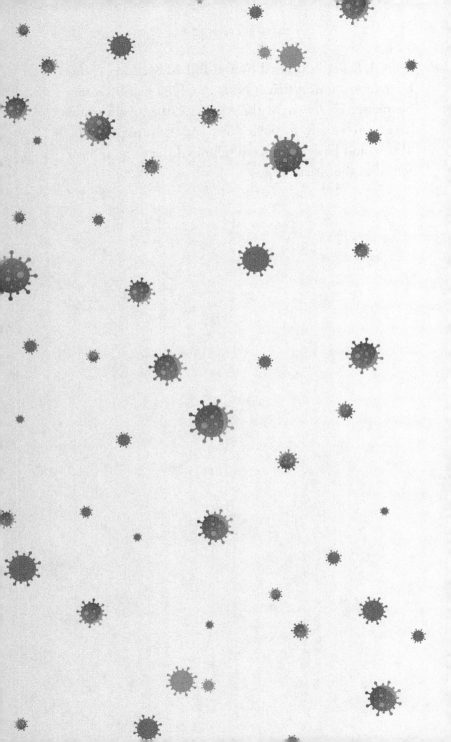

HOW DOES COVID-19 DIFFER FROM OTHER HEALTH OUTBREAKS?

When we think of the major threats to our national security, the first to come to mind are nuclear proliferation, rogue states, and global terrorism. But another kind of threat lurks beyond our shores, one from nature, not humans – an avian flu pandemic.

Barack Obama

THIS SECTION ISN'T meant to be an in-depth history lesson about every viral illness faced by humanity; it is rather a brief overview of the significant outbreaks that the modern world has faced.

The Spanish Flu (H1N1, 1918-1919) infected about 500 million people (one-third of the world's population) and resulted in 50-100 million deaths worldwide.[38,39] This has been among the deadliest events in recorded human history. Unlike today's seasonal influenza, the mortality rate due to the Spanish Flu was high even among young adults (20-40 years of age) rather than primarily among the elderly and infants.[40] This pandemic spread in three large waves: the spring of 1918, followed by a fall wave, and then a winter wave of 1918-1919. The first and third waves were relatively mild. The second wave resulted in millions of deaths.

Although still unclear, some evidence points to the first wave originating from China.[41] The second wave appears to have originated from Southern England. Why was it called the *Spanish* Flu? During World War I (WWI), Allied and Central Powers exercised censorship and covered up news of the flu to keep morale high. Spain, a neutral power at that time, covered the outbreak. Because the Spanish news was the only one reporting on this flu, many believed it had originated in Spain. WWI fueled the pandemic by increasing the contact of different populations who would otherwise be distant. Much like COVID-19, the 1918 pandemic had an enormous societal and economic impact, from shutting down schools and churches to businesses declaring bankruptcy. It was not until the late 1930s and early 1940s when researchers developed the first vaccine for the virus.[42]

The H1N1 and SARS-CoV-2 are both novel viruses in the sense that the world did not have much pre-existing knowledge or immunity, resulting in their dramatic spread. On average, people would show symptoms two days after becoming infected with the 1918 influenza virus.

Most commonly, one infected person would transmit the virus to about two additional people (R_0 1.8). This suggests that the Spanish Flu was less contagious than COVID-19 (median R_0 of 2.79).[43,44]

The Asian Flu (H2N2) emerged from East Asia and spread across the globe from 1957 to 1958. This pandemic resulted in 1.1 million deaths worldwide, with over 100,000 in the US.[45] Similar to the 1918 pandemic, the Asian Flu's second wave resulted in more casualties than the first. The economic disruption was small compared to the prior pandemic, reducing the US' GDP by about 1%. Similar to COVID-19, New York City experienced a higher rate of infections than other cities, and additional physicians were assigned to help treat the surge of patients.[46] No efforts to quarantine individuals, close schools, or cancel large gatherings were made as the US health officials believed such efforts would be futile in disease mitigation. The vaccine was available too late in the pandemic's course to have a meaningful impact. Overall, the Asian flu is considered as a mild influenza pandemic.[47]

The Hong Kong Flu (H3N2, 1968-1970) resulted from mutations in the H2N2 influenza virus about a decade afterward. Originating in China, the Hong Kong Flu resulted in two outbreaks. Interestingly, in the US and Canada, most of the deaths occurred during the first wave (1968-1969), followed by a milder second wave (1969-1970). In contrast, an opposite pattern was observed in Europe and Asia, where the majority of the deaths occurred during the second wave.[48] Although the virus was highly contagious, the strain was even milder than the Asian Flu.

The spread of the virus was accelerated by growth in passenger air travel and as Vietnam War veterans returned to the US. In total, this pandemic resulted in about one million deaths worldwide, including 100,000 deaths in the US.[49] Given the low disease severity and mortality rates in North America, NPIs, such as lockdowns or school closures, were considered unnecessary. In most countries, like the Asian Flu pandemic, vaccines were not available until the pandemic had already peaked.[50]

The Swine Flu (H1N1, 2009-2010) emerged from Mexico after the world had not experienced a pandemic in almost 40 years. Due to globalization and advancements in travel, the Swine Flu spread in six weeks as far as the previous pandemics had in six months. Like the other pandemics, the infection was observed in waves. In the US and Canada, a spring-summer wave was followed by another one in the fall-winter period. In Europe, a mild wave was present in the spring-summer time that was followed by a larger wave in early autumn, which coincided with the reopening of the schools.[51] This pandemic claimed 151,700 to 575,400 lives worldwide.

Most people developed symptoms within two days of acquiring the infection. The duration of symptoms for most was for about six days, and most recovered by nine days after their symptoms began.[52] The US, the UK, and Australia did implement school closures. Overall, the pandemic's economic impact in affected countries was a loss of 0.5-1.5% of their GDP, keeping in mind that a global financial crisis was also unfolding during this period. This outbreak also marked the first pandemic response combining both vaccination and antiviral use.[53]

Severe Acute Respiratory Syndrome (SARS, 2002-2003), similar to COVID-19, originated from a wet market in China. Symptoms usually occurred four-to-five days after being infected, slightly earlier when compared to COVID-19 (five-to-six days).[54] As far as contagiousness goes, one person, on average, infected three others when NPIs were not implemented. With the utilization of public health interventions, one infected person transmitted the virus to less than one more individual.[55] SARS infected more than 8,000 people worldwide and resulted in more than 700 deaths. Overall, 11% of people infected with the virus died as a result of the disease.[56]

Middle Eastern Respiratory Syndrome (MERS) originated from Jordan in 2012. The largest MERS outbreak outside of the Middle East occurred in South Korea in 2015. A few sporadic cases have been reported in Europe, North America, and Africa. On average, symptoms appeared five days after becoming infected.[57] This coronavirus has infected more than 2,400 people worldwide and killed 858. Overall, 34-37% of the people diagnosed with

MERS have died due to the infection.[58] It has alarmingly high fatality rates compared to SARS, COVID-19, or the Spanish Flu. Luckily, MERS is not considered very contagious (R_0 <1) – one infected person transmitted the virus to less than one additional person. However, outbreaks in healthcare settings do show higher infectivity.[59]

Ebola Virus Disease initially appeared as an outbreak in 1976 and then reemerged over 20 times in sub-Saharan Africa. Unlike other diseases, Ebola is not related to influenza or a coronavirus. It is from the virus family of *Filoviridae*. It first emerged as two simultaneous outbreaks from the Democratic Republic of Congo (DRC) and Sudan. The largest outbreak (2014-2016) started from West Africa in Guinea and then spread to Sierra Leone and Liberia. This resulted in more than 28,000 people becoming infected and more than 11,300 deaths.[60] A more recent outbreak, beginning in August 2018, occurred in DRC and was declared a public health emergency of international concern by the WHO in July 2019. This outbreak, which is ongoing at the time of this writing, has been the second-largest ever recorded, with more than 3,400 infections and more than 2,000 deaths.[61] Civil unrest resulting in violence towards Ebola treatment workers has worsened the containment and treatment efforts.[62] Although the outbreaks have primarily been endemic to the African continent, rare cases in other countries such as the US and Russia have also been observed in the past.

Fruit bats are thought of as natural hosts for the virus, infecting humans through intermediate hosts such as chimpanzees and antelopes. Human-to-human transmission is through direct contact with bodily fluids (such as blood or vomit), mucous membranes (nose and mouth), or a broken skin barrier.[63] The most common presenting symptoms include fever, fatigue, and lack of appetite. Less commonly, diarrhea and vomiting, as well as internal and external bleeding (for example, from the gums or rectum) also occurs. Patients usually developed symptoms 8-11 days after becoming infected. Compared to all other infections we have discussed, Ebola is considered the most fatal. Overall, 51% of the people who were infected died due to the virus.[64] Luckily, we have vaccines. A vaccine for Ebola was prequalified in November 2019 and has been used to immunize more than 230,000 people.[65]

Seasonal influenza causes an epidemic every year – even with widely available vaccinations. Hospitalizations and deaths are mainly being seen in high-risk individuals. Influenza causes about three-to-five-million cases of severe illnesses every year throughout the world, resulting in 290,000 to 650,000 deaths.[66] Most people develop symptoms one-to-two days after becoming infected.[67] One person transmits the virus to one additional person (R_0 is 1.28).[68] Seasonal influenza outbreaks generally occur towards the end of autumn and during the winter months.[69]

If millions of people are getting infected every year, why even bother with the vaccine? Because without the vaccine, the number of influenza cases would be considerably higher. The most effective prevention strategy has been vaccination which has been utilized for more than

60 years. Due to the virus' high mutation rates, the vaccines need to be modified every year to match the circulating virus strains. As per the CDC estimates, during the 2017-2018 influenza season, the vaccine prevented about six million infections, 91,000 hospitalizations, and 5,700 deaths in the US alone. Yet not everybody gets vaccinated. During the 2018-2019 influenza season, only 63% of children and 45% of adults were vaccinated. One of the goals of the US government's disease prevention program, known as the Healthy People Initiative, is to increase the percentage of adults and children vaccinated against influenza to 80%.

How do the influenza vaccination rates vary across different countries? For the 2017-2018 influenza season, here is the percentage of people over the age of 65 (the population that is more susceptible to the virus) that was effectively vaccinated: the UK 73%, Canada 71%, the Netherlands 64%, the US 60%, Ireland 58%, Spain 56%, Italy 52%, France 50%, Sweden 49%, and Germany 35%.[70,71,72]

HOW DOES COVID-19 COMPARE WITH SARS AND MERS?

We really need to have a very solid pandemic-preparedness plan and operational capabilities, because this is not something that is going to go away and never happen again.

Anthony Fauci

THE CURRENT COVID-19 pandemic has a lot of similarities to the not-so-long-ago SARS and MERS outbreaks. Various origins of the SARS virus were speculated during the epidemic period. After years of surveillance of SARS-related coronaviruses circulating in a cave in the Yunnan province of China, horseshoe bats' genes were found to be similar to the genes from the SARS virus, which resulted in the human outbreak in 2002. It is now believed that horseshoe bats were the original source of the SARS virus.[73,74] Transmission of the virus has been proposed to be directly from bats to humans or from bats to civets (which are mongoose-like mammals) to humans.[75,76] SARS became the first severe and rapidly transmissible disease to emerge in the 21st century.

When it comes to contagious health outbreaks, timely response from health officials is critical to prevent the spread of the disease and reduce its pandemic potential. So how was the response from the Chinese health authorities during the emergence of SARS? When pneumonia-like cases started emerging in November 2002 from Foshan City in China, the public was kept uninformed about the disease. Until the Ministry of Health announced information about the disease to the public, any physician or journalist who reported on the matter risked persecution by the Chinese authorities. In February 2003, mobile phone messages about a "deadly flu" began to circulate within the region. It was not until February 11, 2003, when the local health officials informed the public and the WHO about the outbreak. On March 15, 2003, more than three months after the start of the outbreak, SARS was declared a worldwide threat by the WHO, and a travel advisory was issued. But by that time, the disease had already spread to Canada, Singapore, Thailand, and Vietnam. After quarantines, travel restrictions, contact tracing, public education, and numerous other efforts, SARS was declared contained in July 2013.

Hospital-related spread of the virus was a prominent feature of both SARS and MERS.[77,78,79] This is likely due to the fact that most of the virus released from a person into the environment (known as viral shedding) occurred only after the person became symptomatic.[80,81] If you're symptomatic, you're more likely to require hospitalization than if you're not showing symptoms. For MERS, almost half to all of the individuals infected were linked to the healthcare setting, and similar observations were reported for some of the SARS outbreaks.[82,83] Similar to the prior coronaviruses, COVID-19 has also shown significant hospital-associated transmission. One study from Wuhan reported that 41% of infections were suspected of having resulted from hospital exposure.[84]

The cost of SARS to the world economy in 2003 is estimated to be USD 40 billion. The impact was more notable in certain sectors of the Asian and Canadian economies. Beyond just the medical expenditures, the heavier toll on the economy was from factors, such as disease prevention measures, the decline in consumer demand (especially in tourism and retail), and loss of foreign investments.[85]

Ten years later, another coronavirus was discovered as the culprit behind pneumonia-like cases. In September 2012, MERS was identified in Saudi Arabia, and similar cases started to appear in other countries, such as Qatar and the UK. When further investigated, the first known cases were determined to have actually occurred in Jordan five months earlier.

MERS, like SARS and COVID-19, has also been found to originate from bats. It is now believed that from bats, the virus was transmitted to dromedary camels, which then infected humans.

Clinically, all three viral infections most commonly result in fever, cough, and shortness of breath. More severe symptoms and poor clinical outcomes are noted in patients of older age and with underlying health conditions.

Interestingly, when hundreds of coronaviruses were studied in cave-dwelling bats after the SARS outbreak, a bat coronavirus (RaTG13) was discovered, which was categorized as low-risk for infecting humans. This strain of coronavirus would further evolve and give birth to the COVID-19 pandemic. Many studies analyzed bat coronaviruses following the first SARS outbreak years before the COVID-19 pandemic. They warned about the potential for reemerging human viral outbreaks arising from bats.[86,87] But unfortunately, our apathetic stance on prevention let COVID-19 emerge unhindered.

5

PERSPECTIVE AS A HEALTHCARE PROVIDER

*He who cures a disease may be the skillfullest,
but he that prevents it is the safest physician.*

Thomas Fuller

S A PHYSICIAN practicing at a university medical center and at a veterans' affairs (VA) hospital in the US, I witnessed how the COVID-19 outbreak affected patient care with newly implemented hospital policies. In anticipation of a surge of patients, more patient beds were added. In March and April, executive orders outlined postponing non-essential procedures and elective surgeries to preserve personal protective equipment (PPE) and healthcare capacity. PPE began to circulate (although, in shortage) among different departments of the hospitals. As non-essential services slowed, many staff members became less busy than usual.

Meanwhile, specific departments, such as the emergency department (ED) and the intensive care unit (ICU), became increasingly busy and even overwhelmed – such as in New York City. As an effort to deal with this shift in patient care, the reassignment of hospital staff members occurred. Nurses, technicians, nursing aides, and even physicians were reassigned to new roles. In an effort to increase the number of frontline workers, some states loosened state licensing requirements and allowed student nurses to enter the workforce early.

SHORTAGE OF PROTECTIVE EQUIPMENT

Leaders across the globe strongly encouraged physical distancing as an effort to minimize human-to-human transmission of the virus. The goal of physical distancing is to reduce new infections, thereby preventing a surge of demand on the healthcare system. This is also termed as "flattening the curve." However, many US hospitals were already reporting shortages of crucial equipment needed to care for their critically ill patients, including invasive ventilators, and PPE for their medical staff. An invasive ventilator consists of a breathing tube which is inserted in a patient's throat and is attached to a machine controlling the patient's breathing. What are the PPE items? PPE usually refers to N95 respirators (masks which seal off the nose and mouth, filtering out 95% or more of airborne particles), surgical masks (which offer less protection than the N95 respirators), goggles, gloves, face shields, wipes and disinfectants, coveralls, and gowns. In April 2020, a survey by a PPE procurement organization found that most institutions had less than two weeks of PPE supplies remaining.[88]

Estimates on the number of invasive ventilators needed to care for the US patients with COVID-19 range from several hundred thousand to a million.[89] Not only do these estimates vary depending on the number, speed, and severity of infections, but interestingly, even the availability of COVID-19 testing affects the number of ventilators needed. Without adequate testing, the number of invasive ventilators required increases. This is because patients who are generally treated with noninvasive ventilators (such as continuous positive airway pressure [CPAP] or bi-level positive airway pressure [BiPAP]) for conditions, such as heart failure or COPD exacerbations, may instead be preemptively intubated while awaiting COVID-19's test results. These conditions which require noninvasive ventilators often present with shortness of breath and cough, mimicking COVID-19 symptoms. Why the preemptive intubation? This is because noninvasive ventilation is not recommended for patients with COVID-19 for fear of an increase in viral particles being released into the air due to pressurized air movement with these machines.

The most recent publicly available data (from 2010) estimated that US hospitals have 62,188 full-feature invasive mechanical ventilators.[90] About 28,883 (46.4%) of these ventilators can be used to ventilate pediatric and neonatal patients. The study also reported that an additional 98,738 ventilators, other than the full-feature mechanical ventilators present, can provide basic functions during a crisis.[91] One study evaluating the outcomes of confirmed COVID-19 patients in China found that 58 of 191 hospitalized patients (30%) required mechanical ventilation. From these patients, 26 required noninvasive ventilation, and 32 needed invasive mechanical ventilation.[92] The US data from New York shows that 12% of patients required the assistance of a breathing tube.[93]

To meet a potential surge in demand, the CDC Strategic National Stockpile (SNS) stores and maintains mechanical ventilators, which can be distributed upon request through appropriate channels. On March 13, 2020, an administrator for the Centers for Medicare and Medicaid Services, reported to CNN that the SNS has between 12,000 and 13,000 ventilators stored. Depending on the size of the incoming surge of patients, various additional factors constrain the capacity of the US healthcare system to provide ventilator therapy. Depending on the influx of patients, limiting factors during a pandemic may include the number of available specialized critical care physicians, bed space with specific functionalities (for example, oxygen supplementation, patient monitoring equipment), and respiratory therapists.[94] A respiratory therapist (RT) is responsible for managing and troubleshooting ventilators, along with administering breathing treatments.

Treatment of patients on mechanical ventilators requires a team of critical care personnel for the best clinical outcomes. This team of personnel includes critical care physicians, critical care nurses, and RTs. Keeping in mind that during a large-scale public health emergency other healthcare workers, such as laboratory technicians (for drawing and analyzing blood samples), X-ray technicians (for performing X-rays), radiologists (for interpreting X-rays and CT scans), and janitorial staff (for cleaning and maintaining patient rooms) will be needed in greater numbers, as well.

HOW TO DECIDE WHO GETS A VENTILATOR?

If the number of patients requiring ventilators surpasses the number of available ventilators, then hospitals and public health officials must consider how to practically and ethically prioritize whom to ventilate.

The principle of *sickest first* is routinely applied to sort patients in the ED, where medical resources are not scarce. Less ill patients will still receive care, but they must wait. For example, a patient with a minor nosebleed will have to wait until a patient with a stroke is taken care of, even if the nosebleed patient was there first. If a pandemic creates a shortage of ventilators, this strategy may lead to more resources being used by patients who, ultimately, may be too sick to survive and fewer resources being available for lesser sick patients who could have benefitted from the ventilators.[95]

The *first-come, first-served* approach has conventionally been used to designate ICU beds during routine, non-pandemic care. Once a patient is being treated in the ICU, they are generally not transferred out if they still need

ICU care (unless the patient or patient's decision-maker agrees to forego life-sustaining treatment). In other words, treating existing patients takes priority over potential benefits to other patients. During routine patient care, the healthcare system can accommodate patients with reduced chances of survival who require ICU beds for days to weeks, yet, who ultimately may not even survive. Others are still able to receive intensive care if needed. However, if ventilators are scarce during a pandemic, these other patients, who may have a much better prognosis if they were to receive intensive care, will not have access to it.

In some situations, in order to use scarce resources most efficiently, those who will probably recover after receiving treatment are given the priority. When treating soldiers with life-threatening injuries, medics give priority to those who are most likely to survive, given a small number of resources. For instance, during cholera epidemics in refugee camps, limited supplies of intravenous fluids are given not to those with the most severe dehydration but instead to those with moderate dehydration who will likely recover with small amounts of fluids.[96]

Historically, from a public health standpoint, decisions to allocate limited resources have been steered by the utilitarian goal of maximizing net benefits. This broad principle can be detailed in multiple ways – for example, maximizing the number of lives saved or maximizing years of life saved. The rule of maximizing the number of lives saved is widely accepted during a public health emergency. This belief is favored from the viewpoint that each life has an equal claim on being saved.

Maximizing years of life saved prioritizes patients who are more likely to have better long-term survival. Let's say we have two patients, Patient A and Patient B, who are both 70 years of age. Patient A only has a medical history of high cholesterol. Patient B, however, has several health conditions, including high blood pressure, diabetes, heart failure, and end-stage kidney disease being treated with hemodialysis. Prioritizing the treatment of Patient A over Patient B will result in more "years of life" saved as Patient B has a significantly shorter estimated long-term survival. This principle is frequently applied in organ transplantation consideration.

Another interesting principle that has been proposed to allocate scarce resources focuses on a person's instrumental value. This refers to an individual's ability to carry out a specific function that is viewed as essential to prevent numerous deaths during a time of crisis. For instance, the federal recommendations prioritize pandemic vaccines to individuals crucial to the pandemic response (for example, public health and healthcare personnel) and to those who maintain essential community services. The rationale is that prioritizing specific key individuals will lead to many more lives being saved through their work.

How do you reach a conclusion regarding the severity of a patient's illness? Over the years, different scoring models have been proposed to help quantify the extent of a patient's disease. One such model, the sequential organ failure assessment (SOFA) score-based triage, was recommended and utilized in some centers during the 2009 H1N1 pandemic. Some parameters assessed by this particular scoring tool include a patient's blood pressure, kidney function, and oxygenation. Other scoring tools, such as acute physiology and chronic health evaluation (APACHE), simplified acute physiology score (SAPS), and mortality in the emergency department (MEDS), have also been proposed and utilized in various settings. When faced with overwhelming demand, a simple triage tool will be useful for the assessment of the sick and facilitate prompt decision making. I do not recommend the use of one scoring tool over another. The healthcare provider should view the available data behind these scores and then decide which fits their patient population and the expected treatment goals.

Any predictive scoring model will not predict the outcome with 100% certainty for any one individual. This concern has limited its use during standard clinical practice. However, the justification for their use is stronger during a severe pandemic when the goal is to maximize outcomes at the population level. The utilization of such an objective approach during a severe pandemic may also be viewed by the public as fairer than decisions based on subjective criteria alone (for example, patient's age, comorbidities). Whichever scoring system is utilized, its performance must be reviewed periodically (ideally during the pandemic) to assess its accuracy and to minimize misclassification of patients' predicted outcomes.[97]

WHO SHOULD MAKE VENTILATOR ALLOCATION DECISIONS?

Separating the roles of clinical care and triage allows physicians to maintain their loyalty to their patients and to act in their best interests.[98] The separation of roles will mean treating physicians will not need to make decisions to withhold mechanical ventilation from patients who require it. Instead, a triage expert (or a triage team) would make such decisions impartially based on the overall outcomes for the population according to predetermined guidelines. Meanwhile, the treating physicians can focus solely on caring for their patients without ethical qualms, within the constraints of the public health emergency.

The role of the triage expert will need to be specified in detail, ideally in advance of the pandemic. Various related factors will need to be considered: required qualifications for the triage expert, establishing necessary training requirements, the protocol for providing support to the triage expert (decisional and emotional support), whether an appeals process will be permitted, and establishment of a system to review triage decisions for quality improvement purposes. The triage expert should be a senior-level provider within the hospital with the experience and authority to implement executive decision-making. A triage team may be more advantageous than relying on a single medical professional. The professional makeup of the team may include a critical care nurse, a respiratory therapist, and a physician. The inclusion of an ethicist (a person specializing in ethical and morally responsible behavior) would be a valuable addition, if available. The triage experts must be chosen based on their past record of trustworthiness, integrity, compassion, competency in making difficult choices, and experience with critical care medicine.[99]

RISE OF TELEMEDICINE

During the 1840s, the telegraph was used during the Civil War to transmit casualty lists and order medical supplies. In the WWI period, radio communication was established, and by 1930, it was used in remote areas, such as Alaska and Australia, to transfer medical information. Current telemedicine systems originated from space-flight programs undertaken by the National Aeronautics and Space Administration (NASA) to monitor the physiological functions of astronauts in space by physicians on Earth. Heart rate, blood pressure, respiratory rate, and temperature were monitored in zero gravity. NASA's experience highlighted the similarity of a physician on Earth trying to monitor, diagnose, and treat an astronaut in space with the needs of a physician trying to diagnose or treat a patient in a remote location here on Earth.[100]

The COVID-19 pandemic led to the rise of telemedicine (healthcare provided via text, audio, or video call) to reduce the transmission of the virus as healthcare facilities could further exacerbate the spread. In general, for chronic and stable diseases (such as heart failure, diabetes, or high blood pressure) management, video consultations tend to have high satisfaction among patients and healthcare staff with similar patient outcomes as traditional clinic visits.[101,102]

Most studies about telemedicine have been performed in patients with stable, chronic conditions. With the emergence of coronavirus and other public health outbreaks, recent studies have analyzed the scope and utility of telemedicine in such settings.

Let's say there are asymptomatic individuals living at home in an epidemic-inflicted location. The individuals, through telemedicine (text or phone/video call), could contact healthcare workers if they start to experience any suspicious symptoms. This would allow for a health assessment, and if the patient's symptoms are concerning, they could be transferred to a referral treatment center. Otherwise, the patient could be periodically monitored at home or advised to seek input from the local primary care physician. During the 2014 Ebola virus outbreak, Guinea's Ministry of Health set up a National Ebola Hotline to respond to public health concerns. It facilitated the referral of suspected cases to a nearby hospital's isolation ward.[103,104] Similar hotlines were set up in Liberia and Sierra Leone, as well.

What about people who are showing symptoms? The use of telemedicine would reduce the exposure time between healthcare workers and infectious patients but still allow for a medical check-up. This would result in a substantial reduction in transmission of the infection through the healthcare channel. A similar strategy was employed in Taiwan during the 2003 SARS epidemic.

Here are a few examples of how telemedicine has been applied within some medical fields:

Anesthesia

In 1974, Gravenstein and his team reported on the use of *laser mediated telemedicine in anesthesia*. They noted that when an anesthesiologist is usually needed in the operating room, the case usually requires general and specific medical expertise rather than manual dexterity. The manual part of clinical anesthesia can be performed by other personnel (for example, nurse anesthetists). The team found that consultants can provide direction to remote staff if the patient and the anesthetizing scene can be viewed on color television. They concluded that telemedicine systems can be successfully employed in the intense and unforgiving environment of an operating room.

For their observations, a two-way system utilizing laser beams was used. The anesthesiologist could view the patient, the anesthetizing area, and the operating room on a monitor and could converse with the other personnel. The system permitted the consultant to pan and tilt the camera, adjust the zoom, and focus by a remote-control panel. Positive clinical outcomes were reported.[105]

Critical Care

Telemedicine has also been used to answer some problems related to the scarcity of critical care specialists. For instance, using a two-way audiovisual link between a small private hospital and a large university medical center, an intensive care specialist provided daily consultations to the smaller hospital. This project showed telemedicine can be a valuable resource linking smaller hospitals to large medical centers and positively influence the quality of care in critically ill patients.[106] These days, ICU telemedicine programs are more widely used and cover at least 11% of ICU patients in the US.[107]

Oncology

In Texas, a telemedicine project to provide oncology consultations to a remote hospital was initiated. The goal was to increase physician contact with the cancer patients and decrease travel expenditures for the oncologists who made monthly visits to the distant hospital. Through the telemedicine system, the oncologists were able to care for their patients through weekly virtual visits rather than on a monthly basis.[108]

Cardiology

The most common cause of death in the US, and in most other countries, is heart disease. Telemedicine has been utilized in the field of cardiology by allowing early (pre-hospital) diagnosis of heart attacks with the electrocardiogram (EKG) transmission. It has also made possible for regular follow-ups of heart failure patients, remotely monitoring and managing devices such as pacemakers and defibrillators, and more. The heart is basically a muscle that pumps blood to the rest of the body. I'm sure you've heard the phrase "time is money." When treating heart attacks, time is muscle. Timely diagnosis and intervention are pivotal to positive outcomes in these patients. Being able to diagnose someone with a heart attack, either on the field or on route to the hospital, is one of the most efficient solutions to reduce the time it takes for treatment.[109]

When might telemedicine not be a good idea? Patients who are severely ill must be assessed in the hospital setting. Also, when a physical examination or procedure cannot be put off for a later time, patients will need to visit the doctor in person.

In general, telemedicine is a promising alternative to in-clinic face-to-face visits in the outpatient care setting. This is particularly important in rural and remote communities (consisting of 50 million people [about 20% of the population] in the US), where a general practitioner may not be available without traveling long distances.[110] Telemedicine has also shown its effectiveness in various public health outbreaks. We are headed into a future of continued telemedicine use combined with in-person visits when necessary. Patients benefit from not having to commute, pay for parking, find a babysitter, and of course, not be exposed to other sick people in the waiting room.

THE QUARANTINE

*Near, far, wherever you are… make sure
you're practicing social distancing!*

Céline Dion

ALTHOUGH ROBUST EFFORTS are underway to develop and stockpile vaccines and antiviral pharmaceuticals, it's unlikely that these measures will be available promptly, and the extent of their effectiveness is uncertain. The initial individual and community containment measures employed in 2020 have been similar to the non-pharmaceutical interventions (NPIs) utilized almost a century ago: isolation of sick people, quarantine of their suspected contacts, physical distancing, simple sanitary measures, such as frequent hand washing and wearing facemasks, and providing the public with information regarding the disease and its risks. Physical distancing refers to maintaining a physical distance of at least six feet from non-household members, as well as limiting activities outside your home.

Essentially, there are two main public health strategies. The first is mitigation, which focuses on slowing (not necessarily stopping) the spread of infection. This is also known as "flattening the curve," thereby reducing a surge of patients and not overwhelming the healthcare system. The second strategy is suppression. This aims to reduce the number of infected people by isolating the sick and practicing physical distancing measures. To augment these strategies, school and university closures are also recommended. The rationale behind this is that children have high contact rates in schools, which favors viral transmission. This is controversial because the number of available healthcare workers absent from work will rise as many will need to stay home to care for their children. It is estimated that about a third of the healthcare workforce have dependent children under 16 years of age.[111] Data from the UK forecasts up to 45% of their healthcare workforce will be absent from work (30% due to school closures, 10% due to illness in staff, and 5% for other reasons). The US models suggest that school closures could lead to 6 to 19% absenteeism of relevant healthcare personnel at the peak of an epidemic.[112] But, this does not take into account other factors, such as the illness of healthcare workers, which would further increase the absenteeism.

How promptly individual countries respond with the implementation of measures, such as NPIs and travel restrictions, is pivotal to the trajectory of their epidemics. In the absence of such interventions, it is estimated that COVID-19 would result in seven billion infections and 40 million deaths worldwide this year.[113]

It is recommended that suppression is maintained until a vaccine becomes available (potentially five years) since it is highly probable that the number of viral cases will rebound when restrictions are loosened. A solution to not remaining under nationwide lockdown for a protracted period of time could be intermittent physical distancing. This would be implemented by trends observed in disease surveillance. Intermittent physical distancing would allow restrictions to be temporarily eased in short periods when infection rates are trending down but could be reintroduced if the number of cases starts rebounding.

LESSONS FROM THE PAST PANDEMIC

The COVID-19 pandemic has resulted in most deaths worldwide since the Spanish Influenza of 1918-1919. Like the Spanish Flu, the economic and the social toll due to the novel coronavirus is considered to be colossal. Many lessons that were learned from the previous major health outbreaks can be applied towards COVID-19. During the Spanish Influenza, only one wave of the epidemic swept over Europe. In the US, however, two surges in the number of deaths were noted a few weeks apart.

Additionally, when compared to Europe, a much more considerable variation in the number of casualties was seen among the US cities. What we have learned from analyzing the past pandemic is that the timing of NPI initiation has a significant effect on the size of the outbreak's wave in different cities. The cities which introduced NPIs early in their outbreaks achieved substantial reductions in overall mortality. For instance, contrast the mortality rates between Philadelphia and St. Louis. In Philadelphia, authorities initially downplayed the seriousness of the Spanish Flu and allowed large public gatherings (for example, a parade on September 28, 1918). School closures and physical distancing interventions were not enforced until the disease had already begun to overwhelm public health resources. During its peak in October, there was approximately one new influenza case every 90 seconds and one flu-related death every 15 minutes.[114] The ongoing WWI (July 1914 – November 1918) had depleted doctors and nurses away to the battlefields, leaving many communities desperately shorthanded. Take East Brady, a town in Pennsylvania, for instance. It found itself with more than three hundred cases of the flu and only one doctor to treat them.[115]

On the other hand, when the first influenza cases emerged in St. Louis, physical distancing measures were promptly put into effect after two days. When measured from their first reported cases, the difference in the response time between the two cities was about 14 days. St. Louis' promptness resulted in one-third fewer deaths due to the Spanish Flu when compared to Philadelphia's sluggish reaction. We learn that if NPIs are successfully implemented early in the epidemic's trajectory, they result in fewer infections. However, this leaves a large population vulnerable to a second wave of infections once interventions relax, particularly if they are lifted too early. In the absence of an effective vaccine, pandemics may have two phases: the first phase being mitigated by NPIs and a second phase occurring as NPIs are eased.[116,117]

UTILIZING NON-PHARMACEUTICAL INTERVENTIONS

If left unmitigated, the pandemic is estimated to result in 2.2 million deaths in the US and 510,000 deaths in Great Britain. During its peak, the demand for ICU beds may exceed by 30 times the maximum capacity of either of these two countries.

Based on the current models, the optimal scenario may still result in eightfold higher peak demand on critical care beds above the available maximum capacity in both the US and Great Britain.[118] This is what happens: if you have fewer hospital beds, a surge in the number of cases leads to more people dying due to the lack of adequate medical care. This forces governments to impose stringent measures, including lockdowns and the closure of businesses deemed non-essential - which further drives down the economy. Therefore, investing in an increase of hospital capacity, distribution of reliable testing, as well as vaccine development, will not only save many lives but will also help ease our economic crippling.

How can we strategically utilize NPIs to suppress the transmission of this virus? First, case isolation at home. This means that people with symptoms must stay at home for at least 10-to-13 days since their symptoms first started. Then, they may break quarantine if their symptoms are gone, they have been fever-free for at least three days, and if testing is available, they have had two negative tests at least 24 hours apart. Asymptomatic patients must practice isolation for 10 days after testing positive. Second, if one member of the household has COVID-19, all household members should remain quarantined at home for 14 days after the last contact with the infected person. Third, the entire population practices physical distancing. Fourth, schools and universities are closed with classes taught through an online platform. Using all four of these methods is estimated to create the best-case scenario and the most substantial impact on the spread of the virus. Such measures will drastically reduce ICU requirements.

But a suppression strategy such as this will need to be maintained for months to years until we have an effective vaccine to prevent a rebound in the number of cases. There is a possibility of an alternative approach to a long-term, nationwide lockdown. That is an adaptive, hospital surveillance-based strategy in which physical distancing and school/university closures may be implemented when weekly new COVID-19 cases in regional ICUs exceed a certain threshold. When the number of new ICU cases fall below a predetermined mark, then physical distancing and school closures can be relaxed, while other NPIs (case isolation, household quarantine) are continued. Depending on the size of the country, this strategy could be utilized nationwide or at the state/provincial level.[119]

IMPACT ON SCHOOLS

As the virus pushes many adults into hospitals and shuts down businesses, it also exiles 1.5 billion schoolchildren out of their classrooms worldwide. This not only disrupts the children's learning but for many, it also results in loss of vital nutrition.[120] In the US, for instance, more than 20 million children from low-income communities depend on the US Department of Agriculture's school lunches distributed for free each day as part of welfare services.[121] As far as children's susceptibility to the infection, based on our current available evidence, children appear to be mostly asymptomatic or have only mild symptoms from the disease. Therefore, the primary rationale behind school closures is to prevent viral transmission from children to their adult household members.

As parents will now have to take care of their children at home, many adults' work capacity and earnings will be restricted. But, do school closures actually reduce viral transmission and people getting sick from COVID-19? If we look at the studies from previous influenza outbreaks, then the answer is yes. However, there is a scarcity of data on the benefits of school closure from coronaviruses (SARS-CoV-1, MERS-CoV, SARS-CoV-2). We then turn to influenza data to help guide decision-making.

What we find is that during influenza pandemics, implementing timely school closures delays and reduces the epidemic peak along with reducing the total number of infections.[122,123]

TESTING AND THE RACE
FOR A VACCINE

I think 50 years from now, people are going to be reflecting historically on [COVID-19] the way we used to reflect on the 1918 outbreak.

Anthony Fauci

TESTING FOR COVID-19 plays a crucial role in our understanding of the disease process, assists with contact tracing, and guides our policymakers on the best course for reopening businesses. The two types of tests which are needed are viral tests and antibody (serological) tests. The viral test informs whether a person has an active infection. An antibody test indicates if the person has been infected in the past.

A viral test, for example, a nose or throat swab, is a two-step process. The first step is obtaining a sample from an individual (for example, swabbing the back of the nose). The second part is amplifying parts of the virus' DNA (viral markers) through Real-Time Polymerase Chain Reaction (RT-PCR). The first step is cheap and easily performed. But, the second part is where our current testing capabilities are limited. Scaling up the capacity for SARS-CoV-2 testing will take time. At the time of this writing, the US is producing 1.2 million tests per week (for a population of 330 million), Germany is producing 500,000 tests per week (for a population of 84 million), and France is producing 210,000 tests per week (for a population of 65 million). Current test production levels are insufficient for mass testing, and each COVID-19 test must be viewed as a scarce, precious resource to be used as efficiently as possible.[124]

One unusual testing method, group testing, has been proposed for specific scenarios. In group testing, samples from multiple individuals can be tested with a single test. If the combined sample test is negative, then that group of individuals is perceived as virus-free. Whereas a positive result indicates that at least one person in the group is infected, without indicating the identity of that person. Group testing has been utilized in the past for syphilis, hepatitis B, and HIV detection. At the writing time, group testing for SARS-CoV-2 has already been implemented in Nebraska and Israel. Testing groups with a similar likelihood of being infected, for example, people working in the same production unit, would result in more efficient testing.[125]

An antibody test detects antibodies. Antibodies are proteins produced by the immune system to help fight infections. Specific antibodies would be present if a person has been infected with the virus and can take one to three weeks to appear. In essence, this test detects a past infection. Antibodies may mean a person has some immunity to the virus. One thing to keep in mind is that during the early phase of an infection, the human body has not produced enough antibodies to be detectable, generating a negative test result even when the person is actually infected. Thus, antibody tests must not be utilized to diagnose active infections.

WHAT MAKES A TEST EFFECTIVE?

All lab tests have some margin of error; however, every test is assessed based on its *sensitivity* and *specificity*. An antibody test, for example, must be *sensitive* enough not to miss present antibodies. Let's say a test has 60% sensitivity. This means the test will wrongly clear 40% of people being tested as not having the disease (false negative). At the same time, the test must be *specific* enough not to mistakenly yield positive results when the person, in reality, does not have the antibodies (false positive). For example, perhaps antibodies of another viral illness, such as influenza, might register positive with the new test trying to assess for COVID-19 and mistakenly identify a person as having had coronavirus. The occurrence of a disease in a population also influences test results. A negative test result may be considered useful and accurate in a population where the infected cases are low – for example, Alaska. However, a negative test result in New York, the US state with a very high number of infections, is more likely to be falsely negative and less useful.

As antibody response to the virus is still being investigated, preliminary data suggests that although IgA and IgG can both be used for antibody testing, IgG remains detectable longer and, therefore, would be preferred for surveillance. IgG can be reliably detected in the second week after disease onset. Additionally, antibody levels are found to be higher in patients with severe infections as compared to patients with mild ones.[126]

Mass reliable testing would allow for individuals who test negative to return to work in strategic sectors of the economy, minimizing a rebound in viral transmission. At the time of writing, we do not know yet if a person who has already been infected with the virus and has developed antibodies is immune from reinfection. Also, if the person is immune, how long does that immunity resist reinfection? With further developments in antibody testing, many answers to the virus' spread and immunity will be easier to answer.

On March 12, 2020, the US Food and Drug Administration authorized the Switzerland-based biotech company – Roche's Elecsys® Anti-SARS-CoV-2 antibody test under Emergency Use Authorization (EUA). The EUA allows for unapproved medical products to be used in an emergency when there are no other adequate or available alternatives. Elecsys® was the first commercially available test to receive the US's authorization for COVID-19.

This is an antibody test, so by analyzing a blood sample, it can help determine whether a person has been previously infected. Roche declares its test to be 100% sensitive and 99.8% specific if the blood is tested 14 days after the onset of infection. This means that if you caught the virus two weeks ago, there is a 0% chance of this test misclassifying you as not having had the disease. The 99.8% specificity means that one in 500 people will test positive for infection without actually having had the disease. Roche also stated that based on their experiments, this test will not falsely result positive for the four coronaviruses known to cause the common cold in humans – making the test more accurate. A single test takes 18 minutes to produce the result.[127] One thing to keep in mind is that since this is an antibody test, it becomes less useful if performed earlier in the disease course – for example, two days after being infected. Compared with the accuracy of other available antibody tests at this time, Elecsys® appears to be in the lead. However, as different tests start becoming available, and we obtain additional data, policymakers will be in a position to choose which tests to keep on the market.

VACCINE

First of all, what is a vaccine, and how does it work? In general, vaccines are comprised of parts of viruses or bacteria, which triggers the body's immune system to make antibodies against that particular germ. By doing so, the immune system is primed and ready to attack any such bacteria or viruses it may encounter in the future. Vaccines tend to be the most cost-effective strategy against infectious diseases – preventing premature deaths and disability. According to the WHO estimates, at least 10 million deaths were prevented between 2010 and 2015 due to vaccinations worldwide.[128,129]

There are four main types of vaccines: inactivated, live attenuated (weakened), subunit/conjugate, and toxoid vaccines. Live vaccines contain live, but weakened, germs to create a robust, long-lasting immune response. The measles, mumps, rubella (MMR) vaccine is an example of a live vaccine. An inactivated vaccine is made from a killed germ to stimulate an immune response. Inactivated vaccines always require multiple doses. Hepatitis A vaccine is an example of an inactivated vaccine. Subunit/conjugate vaccines use a protein or a carbohydrate of the germ to induce a protective immune response. The shingles vaccine is an example of a subunit/conjugate vaccine. Lastly, toxoid vaccines use the germ's modified toxin (toxoid) to elicit immunity – for example, the tetanus vaccine.[130,131]

As governments and pharmaceutical companies accelerate vaccine development efforts, it is important not to prioritize hastiness over safety and effectiveness. There are currently no vaccines against any of the human coronaviruses. Vaccines tested against another coronavirus known to cause infections in cats were found to actually *increase* the cats' development of the disease.[132] Some vaccines for Dengue and the Zika virus have also been reported to generate antibodies, which increase the risk of getting the infection.[133] The effectiveness and safety of a vaccine first have to be tested on animal models and then healthy human volunteers. The reason why vaccine development tends to be more time consuming than producing an antiviral medication is that vaccines are given to healthy individuals.[134] What if, due to a lack of rigorous testing, a vaccine is used on thousands of people and then found to negatively affect the immune system and actually increase the risk of acquiring COVID-19? How will the vaccine affect people who have weak immune systems, to begin with, or patients who are chronically on high dose steroids or chemotherapy (which also weaken the immune system)? Questions such as these must be answered before widespread vaccination is implemented.

Another aspect to be considered is that viruses can mutate. What if the SARS-CoV-2 strains we target with vaccines and antivirals today mutate and exhibit resistance one year from now? The flu vaccine, for example, is modified every year to target the newly mutated, different strains of the virus.

The Chinese authorities shared the virus' genetic sequence with the WHO on January 12, 2020, sparking worldwide research and development for a vaccine. Most of COVID-19's vaccine development is taking place in North America (46%), followed by China (18%), and Europe (18%). The average vaccine requires about 10 years of research and development and costs USD 200 to 900 million.[135,136] At the time of this writing, there are two candidate vaccines in clinical evaluation and 60 candidate vaccines in the pre-clinical phase. The daunting task of vaccine development will require time, funding, and now more than ever, coordinated global efforts. From research and development to data sharing, trials, and then distribution, governments, universities, and pharmaceutical companies must work together.

Given the high likelihood that vaccine supplies will be very limited, at least initially, during a pandemic, various recommendations regarding the prioritization of these scarce resources have been proposed. For instance, the National Vaccine Advisory Committee (NVAC) and the Advisory Committee on Immunization Practices (ACIP) have tier-based recommendations for the dissemination of pandemic influenza vaccines. These recommendations prioritize healthcare workers and vaccine manufacturing personnel. You definitely want the people making and administering the vaccine to not get sick and stick around to be able to help the rest of the population. Next in line will be the highest risk individuals, such as patients older than 65 years of age, with at least one high-risk health condition. Lastly, healthy individuals aged 2 to 64 years without any high-risk health conditions would be considered after prioritizing the other populations.[137]

EFFECT ON THE ECONOMY

Emergencies have always been necessary to progress. It was darkness which produced the lamp. It was the fog that produced the compass. It was hunger that drove us to exploration. And it took a depression to teach us the real value of a job.

Victor Hugo

THE WORLD HAS been struck by a second economic turmoil in just over a decade. But this time the economic downturn has not been caused by a crash in the housing market but by a virus. To prevent an economic collapse in the US, the federal government provided relief packages to combat the 2007-2009 recession. These relief packages, signed by Presidents Bush and Obama, provided billions of dollars in aid. Measures such as cutting taxes for individuals and businesses, creating jobs by funding teachers' salaries and infrastructure projects (for example, transportation, building improvements), and subsidizing healthcare costs were utilized.

On March 6, 2020, the first bill to combat the pandemic, The Coronavirus Preparedness and Response Supplemental Appropriations Act 2020, was signed into law by President Trump. It allocated USD 8.3 billion to improve telehealth availability, enable vaccine development, provide diagnostics and therapeutics, support public health agencies to curb the spread of the virus, facilitate international efforts to assist with the outbreak, and a few other areas. A week later, the US declared a national emergency to tap into USD 50 billion in federal resources to further combat the disease.

The second relief package, the Families First Coronavirus Response Act (FFCRA), was signed into law on March 18th. It allocated USD 3.4 billion to aid employees in receiving paid sick leave, paid family leave to care for children at home due to school closure or to care for a quarantined individual, food assistance, COVID-19 testing, and state unemployment assistance.

On March 27th, President Trump signed the third and the "single-biggest economic relief package in American history" of USD 2 trillion passed by the House and the Senate. The legislation, known as the CARES (Coronavirus Aid, Relief, and Economic Security) Act, aimed at softening the pandemic's blow. It included direct payments for citizens, unemployment benefits, loans for hard-hit corporations, as well as grants and loan forgiveness for small businesses. It also included funding towards healthcare, vaccine development, the building of national stockpile of ventilator and PPE supplies, and other areas.

Although borrowing for public health and financial aid is necessary at times, such as these, the elected officials must remain cautious against wasteful spending. As more and more government finances get pumped into the economy to keep it buoyant, the US is pushed further into debt. The Committee for a Responsible Federal Budget (CRFB) projected deficits of more than US $3.8 trillion for 2020. This was before the USD 484 billion supplement funding to the CARES Act on April 24, 2020, and did not take into account further spending, which is almost inevitable.

THE FEDERAL DEFICIT

What is a federal deficit? Basically, it means that the country is spending more money than it's producing. The government generates finances through taxes and fees or borrows it by selling Treasury bonds, Treasury bills, etc. It spends money on programs such as Social Security, healthcare, and the military. The buildup of each year's deficit leads to the national debt. But why should we care about the national debt? Growing national debt may lead to consequences such as higher taxes and higher interest rates — making it tougher for individuals to borrow money for homes, car payments, or college tuition.

Overall, given our current situation, doing less would undoubtedly do more harm. Without the relief packages, an economic plunge would be inevitable. A recession, or even worse, a depression, would be much more detrimental for the government's fiscal health. If the economy grows at the end of the crisis, the federal debt is manageable. As one of the CRFB directors stated, "When your farm is burning, you don't worry if you have enough water to make it through the next three crop seasons. You put out the fire and then worry about it later."

The US is currently experiencing record-high unemployment rates, a shaky stock market, and a shrunk gross domestic product (GDP). Collaboratively, they signal a potential economic recession. First of all, what is a recession? A recession is a period of falling economic activity lasting more than a few months, which is reflected in the GDP, income, employment, industrial production, and wholesale/retail sales.[138] How long do recessions last? According to Capital Group's analysis of 10 cycles since 1950, these economic downturns have ranged from 8 to 18 months, with the average recession lasting about 11 months.

NOT ENOUGH SUPPLY AND NOT ENOUGH DEMAND

This pandemic began as a supply shock: an unexpected event suddenly changing the supply of a product resulting in an unanticipated change of price. The current global economy is more interdependent than ever before. An item such as a car or a computer consists of parts manufactured all over the world, and cross multiple borders before the final assembly. In January 2020, Chinese manufacturing plants shut down as a response to the virus, creating disruption in the supply chain. As the virus started to spread to the Western countries, the crisis turned into a demand shock. There was a significant reduction in the travel demand, dining at restaurants, and shopping for non-essential items as travel restrictions and lockdowns ensued. China is the world's factory. It makes just about everything. Things such as the popular Ray-Ban sunglasses and the American classic Barbie dolls to the ubiquitous Apple products are all made in China. It's the largest exporter of computer devices, cellphones, and textiles in the world. No other country even comes close to the amount of cement China produces every year. Roads, schools, hospitals, housing, bridges, dams – almost all construction depends on cement. Unsurprisingly, the suspension of manufacturing in China affected many other countries reliant on their factories.

The decreased production of goods as factories shut down (supply shock) and people not paying for items such as restaurant meals, flights, hotels, etc. (demand shock) can cripple specific sectors of the economy. Certain industries, such as transportation, are likely to experience demand shock higher than supply shock. Other sectors, such as mining and manufacturing, are expected to experience larger supply shock relative to the demand shock. Entertainment sectors, restaurants, and hotels experience huge supply and demand shocks, with the demand shock dominating.

Similar to how the average adult catching the SARS-CoV-2 virus has mild and bothersome symptoms for a week or two, most world economies will likely suffer an unpleasant but a short-lived recession. The list of nations with the maximum number of COVID-19 cases, at the time of this writing, is almost identical to the largest economies of the world (with the exceptions of India and Iran). The US, China, Japan, the United Kingdom, France, and Italy are some of the world's top economies and have been most affected by the pandemic. Collectively, the US, China, Japan, Germany, Britain, France, and Italy account for 60% of the world's GDP, 65% of the world's manufacturing, and 41% of the world's manufacturing exports.[139,140] Supply and demand disruptions in these countries will create a ripple effect in the rest of the globe.

There is also a psychological impact of the pandemic on the economy, as previously seen with the 2008 Financial Crisis. Consumers and businesses tend to adopt a "wait-and-see" attitude when faced with massive uncertainty – the type that COVID-19 is now presenting to the world. People and companies tend to postpone purchases and delay investments, which further aggravates the economic impact.

The virus appears to be as economically contagious as it is medically. Many of the world's technology giants are heavily reliant on China for parts and assembly. As an example, United Airlines typically commutes about 50 of Apple's executives between California and China each day. However, it is not the case anymore, as flights to and from China are currently suspended. Analysts estimated that a lack of workers for Apple's manufacturing partner in China would lead to 5-10% fewer iPhones for the first quarter of 2020.[141]

The three significantly impacted COVID-19 areas of Asia – China, Japan, and South Korea, account for over 25% of the US imports and over 50% of the US computers and electronics imports. The origin of the pandemic, the Hubei province of China, is considered the heart of China's "optics valley," home to many businesses producing various components for telecom networks. Potentially a quarter of the world's optical-fiber cables and devices are made there. One of China's most advanced chip-fabrication plants, used to make flash memory used in smartphones, is found there as well.

China is the world's largest automobile market, both in supply and demand. Wuhan, the epicenter of the outbreak and known as one of China's "motor cities," is home to numerous factories supplying automobile parts. General Motors, Nissan, Renault, and Honda are among several companies that have large manufacturing plants in Wuhan. The automobile industry is also being significantly disrupted. Automobile giants such as Volkswagen, Hyundai, Ford, General Motors, and Fiat have temporarily halted production in many of their factories. Disruptions in the supply chain, compounded by a plummeting demand from consumers, resulted in a 79% drop in car sales in February 2020, when compared to the same period last year.

Every day, about 100 million barrels of oil are produced from reservoirs deep below the Earth's surface.

Oil fuels the movement of people and goods around the world. A lot of this has now been halted as governments limit travel and other economic activity to contain the pandemic. ConocoPhillips has delayed drilling in Alaska. Chevron has cut its capital budget for the year by 20%. Many changes are expected as low prices compel firms and governments not just to cancel new projects but to slow their ongoing drilling activities, as well (pun intended).[142]

Crude oil prices plunged into the negatives for the first time in US history. This means that not only was the demand for oil at an all-time low, but companies essentially wanted to pay buyers to take the oil off their hands. Why? The first reason is the decreased global demand. Planes were grounded, and locked-down countries worked from home. Second, there was a storage problem. An excess in the oil supply saturated the storage capacity. Iraq, where 90 percent of the government's revenue comes from oil, will be hit hard as a result.

Shortages in various medical supplies prompted LVMH, the parent company of luxury perfume brands, such as Christian Dior and Givenchy, to begin manufacturing hand sanitizers. General Motors and Tesla are assisting by producing mechanical ventilators. Grocery stores have implemented special shopping hours for the elderly and those with underlying medical conditions. Various companies have donated millions to aid in the pandemic.

Which rising trends in businesses will prosper? For many people, digital payments, working remotely, and e-commerce will outlive the pandemic and become the new norm. Probably, we will see a higher implementation of robotics in factories, replacing many humans and further automating the workplace. Machines cannot transmit lethal viruses to humans.

According to the estimates by JPMorgan Chase economists, the current COVID-19 pandemic is expected to deprive the global economy of more than USD 5 trillion of growth over the next two years. They also estimate that the GDP in developed markets will rise to pre-pandemic levels in the third quarter of 2021.[143]

UNEMPLOYMENT

In April 2020, the unemployment rate in the US hit a record high of 14.7%.[144] That's more than 23 million people. For comparison, the unemployment rate in April 2019 was 3.6%. By the end of April, more than 30 million workers in Europe's largest economies (Germany, France, the UK, Italy, and Spain) had turned to the state for support in wages.[145] Many are comparing the pandemic-related unemployment tsunami to the Great Depression of the 1930s. For the US, the unemployment rate during the Great Depression peaked at 24.9% in 1933, as compared to the rate of 3.2% four years prior.[146] More recently, during the Great Recession (December 2007 – June 2009), the unemployment rate peaked at 10% in the post-recession period. In the US, states with the highest jobless rates were Nevada, California, and Michigan.[147] Outside of North America, France, Italy, the UK, and Sweden had some of the highest unemployment rates in the industrialized nations. While in theory, the recession ended in June 2009, worrying unemployment rates continued until the end of the year.

The COVID-19-driven joblessness also affected some states more than others. At the time of this writing, the states with the highest unemployment rates are Nevada (28%), Michigan (23%), and Hawaii (22%).[148] Nevada and Hawaii being inflicted this vigorously is understandable. Efforts to contain the spread of the virus have led to people staying at home and not going out gambling or snorkeling among other potential virus-carrying people. But, why Michigan? Manufacturing remains Michigan's most profitable industry, led by the production of automobiles and parts. Due to the closures of non-essential businesses, many of the factory workers were sent home and forced to rely on unemployment benefits.

One thing that needs to be considered is that anyone can file an initial unemployment claim, even if they are not eligible. This can lead to falsely high estimates. What needs to be monitored is the number of continued claims (also referred to as insured unemployment), which reflects the number of unemployed workers actually receiving the benefits. This provides confirming evidence of the direction of the US economy.[149] In March 2020, the president of the Federal Reserve Bank of St. Louis, Jamel Bullard, estimated the US unemployment rate could hit up to 30% in the second quarter of the year.[150]

A survey of almost 5,000 US adults in April 2020, conducted by the Pew Research Center found that, from a financial standpoint, lower-income individuals are being impacted more heavily. They are now even more unlikely to be able to pay their bills in full and only 23% of them had enough emergency funds to cover three months of expenses. COVID-19's financial strain was also found to vary across different ethnicities. The results showed that 61% of Hispanics stated that they or someone in their household has experienced a job loss or taken a cut in pay because of the pandemic. In comparison, 44% of blacks and 38% of white adults reported such experiences.[151] In March 2020, Goldman Sachs surveyed more than 1,500 small businesses across 48 states. From these businesses, 51% of them stated that they will not be able to operate for more than three months as a result of the pandemic.[152]

DECLINE IN SALES

Per the US Census Bureau, retail and food service sales in March 2020 dropped by 8.7% compared to the previous month's sales and are lower than March 2019's sales by 6.2%. The previous record drop for any month was a 3.8% fall in November 2008. The decline in retail sales was led by clothing, which went down by 50% in sales compared to February 2020. Furniture sales dropped by 27%, restaurant sales by 26%, and motor vehicle and parts sales by 26%. On the other hand, as individuals stocked up for the lockdown, grocery store sales actually went up by 27% when compared to February 2020.[153]

The US manufacturing output declined in March 2020 by 6.3%. The most substantial reduction in output was in the motor vehicles and parts sector. Total industrial production fell by 5.4% in March 2020 as the pandemic forced many factories to suspend their operations. This has been the steepest decrease in industrial output and manufacturing since 1946.[154] "The collapse in manufacturing output was much bigger than the 3.5% drops in September and December 2008, the worst months of the Great Recession," said Ian Shepherdson, chief economist at Pantheon Macroeconomics.[155]

During the SARS outbreak in 2003, China accounted for 4.3% of the global GDP. Today, China contributes to 16.3% of the world economy.[156,157] Because of this and many other factors, it makes sense that COVID-19 will have a much greater impact on the global economy compared to the SARS outbreak.

The financial strain of a disease results from more than the consequence of the disease itself for the affected people – a pandemic such as COVID-19 influences perceptions and behaviors of many people tied to the economy. For example, let's say a teacher gets infected with tuberculosis (TB). Her TB will cost her (or her government) not only the price to diagnose (chest X-rays, blood tests) and treat (antibiotics) her illness but additional indirect costs, as well. If she is too ill to work, she forgoes her income. If she is considered contagious, she will have to be in isolation for some time, and she will again forgo her income. If she dies due to her new illness, she loses the years of income she would have earned if she were alive. You get the idea.

Similarly, on a larger scale, a disease like COVID-19 would have a much more significant impact on the economy. Not only would you factor in the number of canceled tourist trips and declines in the retail trade, but also numerous other elements because there are links within economies, across various sectors, and across economies in international trade. An economic shock to one country is quickly spread to other countries through the increased business and financial ties associated with globalization. Given the recent events, let's say foreign investors expect further future epidemics to break out in China over the next few years. With this perception, not only would they be more reluctant to invest there, but also, they would demand a greater risk premium for investing in such economies. Their forward-looking behavior would have immediate global impacts.

"Financially, 2020 will go down as the worst year in the history of aviation," said Alexandre de Juniac, the International Air Transport Association's (IATA) Director General and CEO. In June 2020, the IATA estimated that the COVID-19 crisis will result in a loss of USD 84.3 billion for the 2020 year, resulting in a 50% fall in revenue as compared to 2019. For 2021, they expect losses totaling nearly USD 16 billion.[158] If there are additional waves of this pandemic (which is very likely), the losses will rapidly escalate when additional travel restrictions and quarantine measures are implemented. In comparison, the 2008-2009 Financial Crisis set the aviation industry back by USD 31 billion. One thing the aviation industry does have going for them this time is cheap fuel. In 2019, jet fuel averaged US $77 per barrel. The forecast average for 2020 is US $36.80 per barrel.[159]

NETFLIX WHEN ILL

When consumers are forced to sit at home, online vendors thrive. Traffic to Netflix's US registration webpage rocketed during March 2020. Outside of the US, where its largest growth targets are, Netflix's usage spiked in countries such as Greece, Italy, and the Philippines. Its growth in users surged as more parts of the world went into lockdown.[160] Certain businesses, such as online merchants and grocery stores, are thriving during this pandemic. The use of Zoom, an online video conferencing platform, has soared as corporations, schools, and other organizations work from home during the lockdown. It went from about 10 million maximum daily users (both free and paid) at the end of December 2019 to 200 million in March 2020.[161]

HOW WILL LOCKDOWN AFFECT VARIOUS COUNTRIES?

Nations that depend on labor-intensive activities and regions with large construction sectors, such as many Central European countries, look vulnerable. The same goes for the countries that rely on tourism – which accounts for one in eight non-financial jobs in Southern Europe. Conversely, nations with more jobs that can be done from home (for example, financial advisors), will likely fare better. Job opportunities that are falling the fastest are occupations hit directly by the virus containment measures. They include hospitality, tourism, personal services, and certain retail services. Countries with a higher percentage of employment in these occupations, such as Ireland and the UK, are seeing some of the largest declines in online job postings on Indeed (an employment search engine). Compared to April 2019's trends, this year, Australia saw a 41% decline, the UK 36%, Canada 36%, Ireland 32%, and the US a 24% decline in job postings on Indeed. The most massive drops in job postings were in beauty and wellness (-80%), hospitality and tourism (-76%), and food preparation and service (-68%).[162]

Assuming countries hit hard by the pandemic lose 8% of their working days this year (due to the lockdown), the International Monetary Fund (IMF) predicts that the global GDP will shrink by 3% for the year 2020. Per the IMF, the US' GDP is expected to reduce by 5.9% and Europe's GDP to contract by 7.5% in 2020. This is assuming the pandemic fades in the second half of the year. So, what are the measures taken by countries to counter these economic hits? As of the end of May 2020, about USD 9 trillion have been deployed by countries throughout the world to help people and businesses fight COVID-19. This includes direct payments to citizens and businesses, postponement of taxes, loans by governments, public operations, etc.[163] As of May 29th, 2020, financial support from the G20 countries has been estimated to exceed 10% of their 2019 GDP.

The elderly face a much higher risk of severe health complications or death if infected compared to the young. At the same time, the cost of reduced economic activity disproportionately affects the younger population more who bear the brunt of lower employment. Due to this, the two age groups will have different views about the optimal mitigation strategy.[164]

The African continent has been relatively spared from the virus when compared to its Western counterparts, at the time of this writing. However, many African countries do appear to be affected by containment efforts utilized by others. The number of poor people in Africa (based on the US $1.90 per day poverty line definition) is expected to increase by 5 to 16%. That's an increase of 59 to 200 million people in poverty due to the pandemic's effect on industrial production, retail sales, and more. East and West Africa would be affected more strongly than the other regions.[165]

HOW MUCH WORK CAN BE PERFORMED FROM HOME?

Data from the US and the UK collected in late-March 2020, delineates the number of tasks that can be done from home broken down by occupation. Some occupations, such as those pertaining to business/finance or computers, have a large portion of tasks that can be done remotely (almost 70%). Other industries, such as food preparation or transportation have a tiny percentage of tasks that can be done from home (20%).[166]

Chinese adults in 64 cities were surveyed in February 2020, one month into their lockdown. The surveyors found that 27% of the adults continued to work at the office, 38% worked from home, and 25% stopped working altogether due to the outbreak. Additional factors, such as

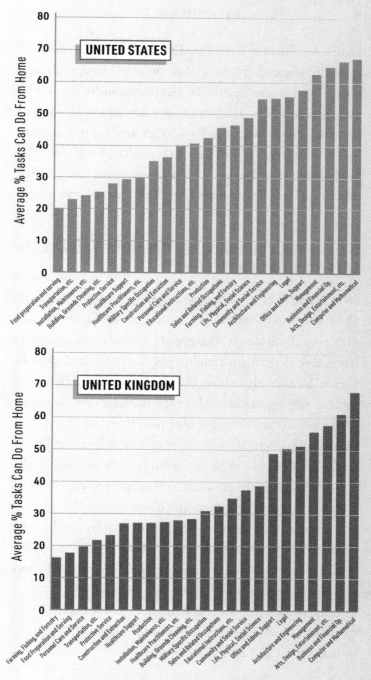

Credit: "The large and unequal impact of COVID-19 on workers", VOX, CEPR Policy Portal

health conditions, as well as distress and life satisfaction, were also assessed. Those who stopped working completely reported worse health. Interestingly, individuals who exercised more than 2.5 hours per day had lesser rates of life satisfaction. Individuals who exercised for half an hour a day or less were more likely to be satisfied with life.[167] It is plausible that the more active group was less satisfied due to the restrictions affecting their exercise routines.

THE HIGHER YOUR INCOME, THE MORE YOU ARE ABLE TO WORK FROM HOME

How are workers in different income distributions affected by the lockdown? As we can see in the figures on the next page, individuals with greater annual earnings report being able to perform a higher portion of their tasks from home. Studies also show that job losses have been the highest among workers who earn the least. For instance, in the UK, from almost 4,000 people surveyed towards the end of March, 16% of the people with incomes below USD 12,600 (£10,000) reported having lost their jobs due to the virus. In contrast, 5% of people experienced job losses in the higher income distribution.[168]

Overall, it appears that 34% of US jobs can be performed from home. However, there are significant variations across different cities and industries. Some of the top metropolitan areas with the highest share of jobs that can be done from home are San Francisco, San Jose, Washington, D.C., and Austin, Texas.[169] More than 40% of jobs in these cities can be done from home.

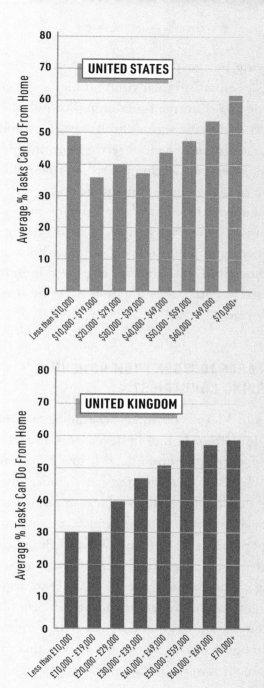

UNITED STATES

Average % Tasks Can Do From Home

Less than $10,000
$10,000 - $19,000
$20,000 - $29,000
$30,000 - $39,000
$40,000 - $49,000
$50,000 - $59,000
$60,000 - $69,000
$70,000+

UNITED KINGDOM

Average % Tasks Can Do From Home

Less than £10,000
£10,000 - £19,000
£20,000 - £29,000
£30,000 - £39,000
£40,000 - £49,000
£50,000 - £59,000
£60,000 - £69,000
£70,000+

Credit: "The large and unequal impact of COVID-19 on workers", VOX, CEPR Policy Portal

Varying by the country, specific industries were deemed "essential" to their communities and were recommended to continue functioning for public health and safety. Industries such as healthcare, food and agriculture, energy, and financial services continued to operate. So, when considering the risk of unemployment if the job cannot be done from home during a country-wide lockdown, the *essentialness* of the job must also be taken into account. For example, most healthcare workers, farmers, and police officers cannot work remotely from home. Still, since they are employed in industries considered essential, they are unlikely to be at risk for unemployment.

WHO IS ABLE TO WORK FROM HOME IN DEVELOPING COUNTRIES?

Only about 13-15% of workers (assuming farming cannot be done from home) in developing countries can plausibly work from home – far below that in the US (34%). However, the estimates vary significantly across different developing countries – for example, 6% of Ghana's population can work from home as opposed to 23% of the population in Yunnan, China.[170] Because of the prevalence of the agricultural sector in rural areas of developing countries, the ability of a farmer to work from home significantly affects the findings. If farm plots are adjacent to the farmer's home, as well as the output is consumed at home and not sold to the market, then farming from home is feasible. If, however, farmers are assumed to have minimal ability to work from home, the gap in work-from-home ability between the rich and poor countries widens further.[171] Interestingly, if it is assumed that most of the farmers can work from home, then the ability to work from home in poor countries (64%) exceeds that of developed countries (38%).[172]

WHY HAS COVID-19 TREMENDOUSLY IMPACTED THE STOCK MARKET?

At first, the answer seems obvious: as more people get ill or are forced to stay at home, there is lesser work being conducted, which negatively impacts the economy. But, looking back at the Spanish Flu's economic impact in 1918-1919, it did not remotely resemble such stock market jumps. A potential answer may be that, compared to the pandemic a century ago, information today is richer and diffuses much more rapidly. This allows for information through the media to influence a much larger population, shaping the beliefs and behaviors of shareholders and investors. Also, today we have much more interconnectedness: a global economy. We see this with the routine intercontinental travel, everyday cross-border commuting (for example, in Europe), falling tariffs, and just-in-time inventory systems (which are highly vulnerable to supply disruptions). The pandemic-stemmed containment policies have extensively dammed the flow of labor to businesses, vastly reducing the output of goods and services.[173]

THE PANDEMIC'S EFFECT ON THE FINANCIAL MARKET

It's estimated that 46% of the firms in the S&P 500 (stock market index that measures the stock performance of the 500 largest companies in the US) included pandemics (or other health crises) as a risk factor to their businesses. Interestingly, from January to March 2020, firms which included pandemics as a risk factor experienced a decrease in value almost equal to the firms which did not include the pandemic as a risk. This suggests managers underestimated their exposure to pandemics and whether firms included pandemics as a risk factor does not correlate with its change in value due to the pandemic.

At the industry level, firms which experienced the steepest decline in value were petroleum and natural gas, apparel, restaurant and hotels, transportation, and automobile. The firms with the largest decline in value at the onset of the pandemic included Norwegian Cruise Lines (-86% change in value), Noble Energy (-83.7%), Royal Caribbean Cruises (-83.4%), Halliburton (-80.6%), and Carnival (-80.5%). A few corporations that increased in value because of the pandemic include Walmart (+0.4%), General Mills (+3.0%), Netflix (+0.6%), Clorox (+26.0%), and Regeneron Pharmaceuticals (+31.2%). Government bonds increased in value, while the S&P Corporate Bond Index decreased in value. The US dollar increased in value as compared to the Euro, GBP (British pound), and Japanese Yen.[174]

PHYSICAL DISTANCING AND BUSINESS

Face-to-face interactions are more common in dense cities. Physical distancing, which includes limiting activities outside of home, imposes disproportionately higher limitations on certain urban sectors such as retail, accommodation and food services, and entertainment. In the developed world, industries such as agriculture and construction are less reliant on face-to-face communication and will be less affected by physical distancing. This knowledge is useful for policymakers to help target fiscal assistance to businesses that will be most disrupted by physical distancing.[175]

WHICH OCCUPATIONS ARE CONSIDERED HIGH OR LOW RISK FOR COVID-19 EXPOSURE, AND WHAT ARE THEIR EARNINGS?

On the next page is an infographic that provides a visual representation of various occupations along with their exposure risks and approximate annual salaries. The exposure risk is calculated based on the occupation's physical contact with others and the job's exposure to diseases. As we can see, one of the jobs with the highest risk would be that of the dental hygienist. On the other hand, economists would have the lowest COVID-19 exposure risk.

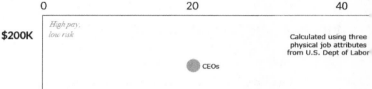

COVID-19 Occupational Risk Score

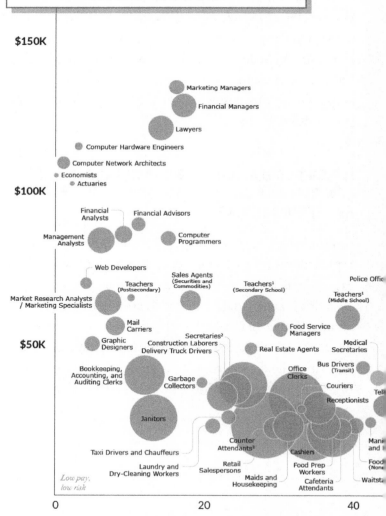

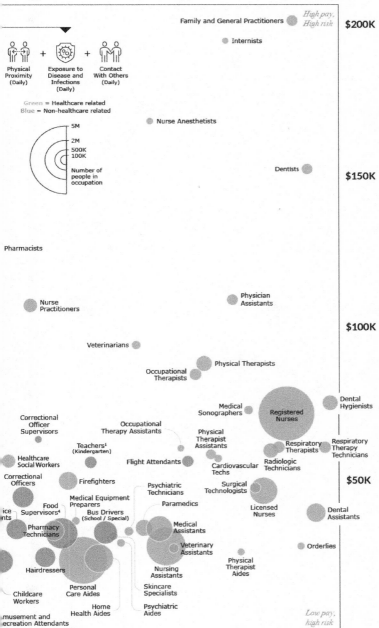

60 80 100

Family and General Practitioners — *High pay, High risk* — $200K

Internists

Physical Proximity (Daily) + Exposure to Disease and Infections (Daily) + Contact With Others (Daily)

Green = Healthcare related
Blue = Non-healthcare related

5M
2M
500K
100K
Number of people in occupation

Nurse Anesthetists

Dentists — $150K

Pharmacists

Nurse Practitioners

Physician Assistants

$100K

Veterinarians

Physical Therapists

Occupational Therapists

Medical Sonographers

Registered Nurses

Dental Hygienists

Correctional Officer Supervisors

Occupational Therapy Assistants

Physical Therapist Assistants

Respiratory Therapists

Respiratory Therapy Technicians

Teachers¹ (Kindergarten)

Flight Attendants

Cardiovascular Techs

Radiologic Technicians

$50K

Healthcare Social Workers

Correctional Officers

Firefighters

Psychiatric Technicians

Surgical Technologists

ice nts

Food Supervisors⁴

Medical Equipment Preparers

Bus Drivers (School / Special)

Paramedics

Licensed Nurses

Dental Assistants

Pharmacy Technicians

Medical Assistants

Veterinary Assistants

Physical Therapist Aides

Orderlies

Hairdressers

Nursing Assistants

Skincare Specialists

Childcare Workers

Personal Care Aides

Home Health Aides

Psychiatric Aides

Low pay, high risk

musement and ecreation Attendants

60 80 100

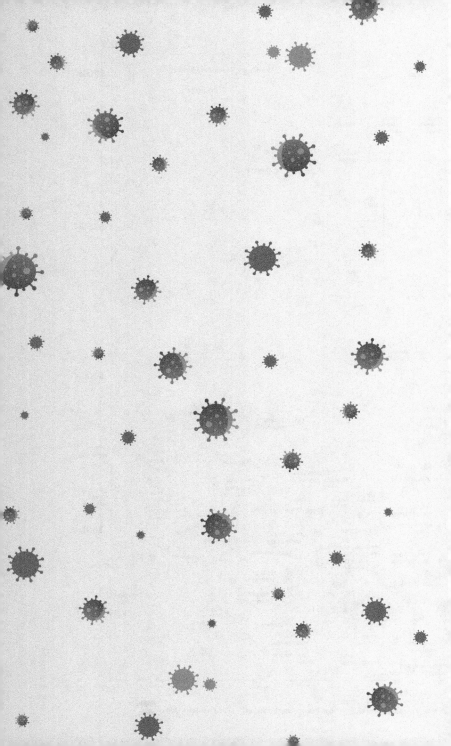

IMPACT ON THE WORLD

*I am not afraid of an army of lions
led by a sheep; I am afraid of an
army of sheep led by a lion.*

Alexander the Great

T STARTED AS a health crisis, which led to an economic crisis and then evolved into a political crisis. In the last two decades, our world has faced many calamities: earthquakes, hurricanes, wildfires, terrorism, economic recessions, and now a significant pandemic that is reshaping society in many ways. COVID-19 may be among the most challenging tests of political leadership that the world has ever seen.

HOW DID DIFFERENT WORLD LEADERS RESPOND TO THE PANDEMIC?

Brazil's right-wing president, Jair Bolsonaro, initially downplayed the pandemic's threat and sabotaged quarantine measures imposed by nearly all of the country's state governors. He urged the citizens to ignore state governors who had ordered lockdowns and physical distancing measures. Why? He believed that shutting down the economy would impair his chances of re-election.[176] His supporters stood by him as he insulted women and racial minorities. But more people started drawing the line at his mismanagement of the pandemic. As the sixth-largest country by population in the world and the largest Latin American country, Brazil was already vulnerable to a swift spread of COVID-19. Not long after, the country found itself overwhelmed with the virus with more than a million cases, and that number continues to rise.

Denmark was one of the first European countries to implement a nationwide lockdown – even before reporting any deaths from the virus within its borders. According to a survey released in April 2020, 86% of the respondents viewed the Danish Prime Minister, Mette Frederiksen, as having handled the pandemic appropriately. Not surprisingly, her polling approval rate went up from 39% in March to 79% in April 2020.[177] One month after the lockdown, Denmark began gradually easing its restrictions. In mid-April, 2020, it was the first country in Europe to reopen some of its schools and then small businesses. The country's prompt preventative lockdown, partly due to its centralized government, has allowed for an early reopening without a spike in its COVID-19 cases.

The UK, with almost 300,000 COVID-19 cases as of June 2020, is one of the most affected nations in the world. Its government has been criticized for a delay in implementing a lockdown and other strict viral suppression measures. On March 10th, 2020, a gathering of more than 250,000 people took place at a horse-racing event in England when no caution against mass gatherings had been relayed to its citizens. One of the UK's most influential advisers on the pandemic stated the country's death toll could have been halved if the lockdown had been implemented only a week earlier. Its leaders have also been blamed for testing and PPEs not being available widely or promptly enough.

On March 11, 2020, the WHO characterized the novel virus as a pandemic. About a month afterward, most world leaders saw a rise in their net approval ratings. Justin Trudeau (Canada) experienced a 19-point rise, Scott Morrison (Australia) a 25-point increase, Angela Merkel (Germany) a 15-point rise, Narendra Modi (India) an 11-point rise, Boris Johnson (UK) a 19-point increase, Emmanuel Macron (France) an 11-point rise, Andrés Obrador (Mexico) a three-point rise, and Donald Trump (USA) a 3-point increase. Unsurprisingly, some leaders saw a decline in their approvals within the same timeframe: Jair Bolsonaro (Brazil) by three points and Shinzo Abe (Japan) by one point.[178]

"Rally-around-the-flag effect" is how political scientists describe a sudden temporary boost in the popularity of leaders during a crisis. Why? One explanation is from the patriotism perspective. Individuals respond to a threat by identifying with their leader. Another reason is the information environment changes because opposition leaders tend to fall silent during a crisis.[179] A similar effect was witnessed after the attacks on September 11, 2001, in the US: Bush's approval rating soared from 51% on September 10 to 90% on September 22, 2001.[180]

Under the leadership of Jacinda Ardern, New Zealand is another example of a nation and its officials handling the pandemic well. In the first week of April, about a month after the WHO declared the outbreak a pandemic, a poll found that 88% of Kiwis (colloquial term for New Zealanders) "trust[ed] the government to make the right decisions on COVID-19." In comparison, 60% of the US, 68% of Great Britain, and 67% of Germany's respondents felt the same about their own leaders.[181] Two days after the declaration of the pandemic in March 2020, New Zealand began canceling mass gatherings. On March 19, 2020, for the first time in history, the country closed its borders to foreigners. This was followed by shutting down public services (libraries, galleries, etc.) shortly after, and after seeing a rising number of cases, a full-fledged lockdown was implemented on March 26, 2020. New Zealand's swift and centrally-planned reaction to the virus has been key to keeping their infection rates low and the death toll to only 22, at the time of this writing. Seeing a decline in the number of new cases, the country began easing some of its restrictions towards the end of April and returned to normalcy on June 9, 2020.[182] Ardern's successful pandemic response is attributed not only to her giving a clear direction but also to providing meaning and purpose to what is being asked from the citizens, and showing empathy. Her leadership has highlighted the success of female leaders during this pandemic, along with other countries led by women, such as Norway, Iceland, Finland, Taiwan, Germany, and Denmark. Perhaps it's time to rethink the macho style of governance popular in many other countries.

In Switzerland, as soon as the first two cases were identified, the government built testing centers and required that large events (more than 1,000 people) be canceled. Expensive exhibitions, such as the Geneva Auto Show and the prestigious watch shows, were instantly canceled.

As nations focus inward to tackle COVID-19, some countries have realized their mischievousness may go unnoticed. The pandemic has allowed power-hungry leaders to illegalize mass protests, postpone elections, silence their opposition, and censor media. On March 30, 2020, a "coronavirus law" issued by Hungary's parliament granted its Prime Minister, Viktor Orban, extraordinary powers without the need to consult with other lawmakers to implement decisions. They justified this as a needed policy to deal with the pandemic and diminish "claim or spread of falsehood." Orban has essentially been empowered to be a dictator. The parliament is able to repeal his powers, but since his party has two-third of the seats, it will probably not happen.[183,184]

We had seen such seize of power in the past when in 2004, Vladimir Putin centralized control over Russia as a response to terrorist attacks. In 2016, a failed coup against Turkey's government led its president, Recep Tayyip Erdogan, to impose a state of emergency. Critics claimed that this new power was used by Mr. Erdogan to target his political opponents with the same authority as suspected coup conspirators.

In April 2020, Cambodia's parliament passed a state of emergency law. This new law empowered its Prime Minister, Hun Sen, to monitor communications, control media along with social media, and restrict information the government believes could cause public fear or unrest.

Crowded jails breed infection. Opponents and critics of some ruling governments understand that voicing their beliefs could lead to detention and risk being infected. Turkey, Europe's second-biggest jailer with about 294,000 inmates, plans to release 45,000 prisoners to minimize COVID-19 transmission, and another 45,000 to be put under house arrest. This reform is highly criticized as this amnesty is not being considered for political prisoners, journalists, and human rights advocates.[185]

HOW DID THE US HANDLE THE PANDEMIC?

The US has the highest number of COVID-19 infections and deaths in the world at this time. The first confirmed infection in the US was on January 20th, 2020. By mid-June, more than two million citizens had been infected, and more than 118,000 were dead because of the virus. At the time of this writing, these numbers continue to grow. For comparison, 58,220 Americans died in battle during the Vietnam War, and 53,402 died in battle during WWI.[186] What this means is that COVID-19 has killed more Americans in six months than the 11-year-long Vietnam War and the four-year-long WWI combined. What a tragedy!

So, what was wrong with the US's response to the pandemic? One important answer is viral testing. Testing for the virus has been crucial to curb its spread in countries like South Korea and Germany. The US was far too slow. In addition to diagnosing and isolating the infected, testing is essential to estimate the trajectory of the pandemic. This allows experts to forecast hospital surges, the number of medical personnel required, ventilator equipment needed, and so forth. Without useful, robust testing data, the epidemiologists' recommendations lean more towards educated guesses rather than informative calculations.

On January 31, 2020, one day after the global health emergency was declared by the WHO, the US announced a suspension of entry of many (but not all) people traveling from China effective February 2, 2020. At the same time, quarantines were also set for Americans who had recently returned from parts of China. Another reason attributed to the mismanagement of the outbreak is the White House downplaying the virus. Initially, majority of the messages from the White House and President Trump continued to deemphasize COVID-19. For instance, on March 9, 2020, Trump compared COVID-19 to the flu: "So last year, 37,000 Americans died from the common flu…nothing was shut down, life and the economy go on. At this moment, there are 546 confirmed cases of Coronavirus, with 22 deaths. Think about that!" At last, on March 31, 2020, he corrected his comparison: "It's not the flu. It's vicious." From blaming the "incompetence of China, and nothing else, that did this worldwide mass killing," on May 20, 2020 to blaming the Obama administration for the country's shortage of testing kits, it seemed as if the Trump administration always had an excuse for the mismanagement of the pandemic.

In April 2020, Trump accused the WHO of "severely mismanaging and covering up the spread of the coronavirus" and suspended the US funding to the WHO, pending a review of its COVID-19 response. The US taxpayers provide USD 400 - 500 million to the WHO each year. The organization was also criticized last year about its reluctance to declare the Ebola outbreak as an international public health emergency. The Director-General of the WHO, Dr. Tedros Ghebreyesus, responded by stating that when raising money for the Ebola outbreak, the donor nations "refrain from paying until there is fear and panic," and recommended more routine funding.

The White House announced a three-phased approach for "opening up America again." They recommended that states wait for a "downward trajectory of positive tests" over a 14-day period. The states that satisfy this criterion can consider cautiously reopening while still maintaining physical distancing, with schools remaining closed, and venues such as movie theatres to operate under physical distancing protocols.[187]

THE PANDEMIC AND POLITICS

COVID-19 has magnified the partisan divide within the US, and the upcoming presidential elections have further vividly highlighted the differences. Republicans are more likely than Democrats to think the Coronavirus threat is exaggerated. A survey of about 4,600 adults in March 2020 found contrasting perceptions on COVID-19. From the responders, 62% of Republicans viewed the seriousness of the pandemic as "generally exaggerated." On the other hand, 31% of Democrats felt the same. Additionally, Republicans were more likely to attend social gatherings in the midst of the pandemic as compared to Democrats.[188]

At the beginning of March 2020, about 1,200 voters were called and inquired about the pandemic. From these voters, 68% of Democrats were either "very concerned" or "somewhat concerned" that they or someone they knew would be infected with the novel coronavirus. In contrast, 63% of Republicans were "not so concerned" or "not concerned at all." Not surprisingly, 87% of Republicans approved of the way Donald Trump was handling the response to the coronavirus as compared to only 10% of the Democrats. Additionally, 66% of all the responders had confidence in the US healthcare system to handle the response to the coronavirus.[189]

COVID-19 quickly spread through the Southern US states. As some Americans, fed up with the lockdown and unemployment, protested that public health officials have infringed upon their "liberty" and "freedom," few of the states began reopening for business at the end of April 2020. Despite warnings from health officials, Georgia and Oklahoma announced plans to partially reopen their businesses in April.[190,191] What makes the Southern US particularly vulnerable to the pandemic is that it has a disproportionate number of uninsured, unhealthy, and incarcerated Americans.[192,193,194] This means the Southern population is not only more likely to contract the disease but also more likely to die when infected – based on what we already know about the COVID-19 mortality demographics. If the COVID-19 outbreak were to spread uniformly throughout the states, West Virginia, Alabama, Mississippi, South Carolina, and Arkansas are considered to be the highest-risk states for severe illness.[195]

BEYOND THE PANDEMIC

*One who conquers the sea today is ready
to conquer the ocean tomorrow.*

Matshona Dhliwayo

AS THE PANDEMIC slowly passes for several countries, in the coming months, governments will start loosening lockdown orders, and more businesses will reopen. In the near future, we can expect significant changes in how we live our everyday lives. Airports and train stations will not have large crowds. Stadiums will be mostly empty. Diminished demand from consumers will result in a gloomy world economy. Undoubtedly, the collaboration between medical researchers, pharmaceutical companies, and governments will be crucial for vaccine and antiviral breakthroughs.

As enormous amounts of resources and time are poured into medical research, the invention of an effective vaccine will make the people safe and the pharmaceutical companies wealthier. We will also likely see breakthroughs in diagnostic medicine. Imagine being able to purchase a test kit from your local pharmacy and test for a viral illness at home, like the convenience of a pregnancy test.[196] We will see increased antiviral medications being developed. This surge in research and development will lead to various unexpected benefits. Let's take a hypothetical scenario: a new antiviral medication against coronavirus is being tested. When tested on humans and its data analyzed, it's found to also decrease the rates of cervical cancer in women. Wait... what? Cervical cancers are generally caused by the Human Papillomavirus (HPV). Intending to prevent the coronavirus from escaping one human cell and entering another, perhaps, the new medication inadvertently also affects the viral replication of HPV. Spin-off benefits, such as this, are actually quite common in the medical realm. For instance, minoxidil (brand name Rogaine) was initially used to treat high blood pressure. Interestingly enough, it was incidentally discovered to cause hair growth and, to this day, continues to be used to treat baldness.

New technologies and medical innovation should, hopefully, prepare us for the next pandemic. With the end of WWII, leaders built international institutions such as the United Nations (UN) to prevent future conflicts and mass casualties. After our pandemic, leaders will prepare international organizations to prevent the next infectious outbreak. Topics such as stockpiling, travel restrictions, social gatherings, hospital preparedness, and international cooperation will be discussed. This will not only prepare us for the next pandemic but will also defend us against potential bioterrorism.

Wealthy nations must include poorer ones in preparedness planning. The pandemic has shown us that viruses don't need passports, and we are all connected biologically by microscopic germs. Even the most self-interested government should agree with this by now. Wealthier nations have to aid poorer ones in developing their primary healthcare systems. If a novel virus appears in a poor country, we want its doctors to be able to identify an outbreak and contain it as soon as possible.[197]

CHANGE IS IN THE AIR

On a more optimistic note, the pandemic is showing positive effects on the environment. Due to the reduction in traffic and transport along with the closure of factories, air pollution has decreased – at least temporarily. From the wide range of air pollutants, fine particles, also known as atmospheric particulate matter with diameters of less than or equal to 2.5 micrometers ($PM_{2.5}$) and nitrogen dioxide (NO_2), are among the most ubiquitous and widely studied indicators used to quantify air pollution. A $PM_{2.5}$ particle is about 30 times smaller than the width of a single human hair. Nose hair can filter out dust and dirt but not $PM_{2.5}$. This allows these microscopic particles to readily move into our lungs and then into our blood.

Breathing in air with high concentrations of $PM_{2.5}$ directly impacts people with respiratory conditions, such as asthma or COPD. But what's even more concerning is that long-term exposure to these fine particles increases the risk of death from heart disease, stroke, lung cancer, and lung infections.

Worldwide, ambient air pollution is one of the most important risk factors for death and disability. In 2016, $PM_{2.5}$ killed more than four million people.[198] That's more global deaths than from some other well-known risk factors such as alcohol use and physical inactivity. Similarly, NO_2 has also been linked to causing various health conditions, such as cancer, heart disease, diabetes, and asthma.[199,200]

In China, changes in the air quality by measurements of NO_2 and $PM_{2.5}$ were studied in 367 cities from January 2016 to March 2020. Because of the Chinese lockdown, significant decreases in NO_2 and $PM_{2.5}$ were observed. The improved air quality during the lockdown period is estimated to have avoided almost 9,000 NO_2-related deaths and more than 3,000 $PM_{2.5}$-related deaths in China.[201] Satellite sensors have revealed an unprecedented NO_2 decline over China, South Korea, Western Europe, and the US as a result of public health containment measures from January to April 2020. In China, NO_2 levels dropped by 40% on average in cities affected by the lockdown. The NO_2 levels also reduced by 28% in New York and by 24% in Philadelphia.[202]

NO MASK, NO SERVICE

So, in what ways can we expect our lives to change as the lockdowns ease? We can expect restaurants to limit the number of diners to half of their pre-pandemic capacity and potential fines for eateries that do not enforce such caps. Social distancing will likely continue to be utilized in various public outlets, from restaurants and grocery stores to banks and movie theatres. Scrupulous hygiene routines will be the norm. Imagine a world where hand sanitizers are strategically placed upon public entrances, workers disinfect tables after usage by each diner, and the widespread usage of masks in public. Contactless payments via smartphones, credit cards, and wristwatches, which eliminate the need to swipe, sign, or tap (reducing the spread of germs), will be prevalent among vendors. We will see more online ordering with either self-pickup or a further increase in delivery services.

How will our flight experience be different due to COVID-19? We will likely see screening measures at airport entrances. A sick passenger spreading the disease will be detrimental to that airline. You'll think twice about purchasing a ticket with a particular airline if you've learned that someone with the virus recently infected others during a flight. You will either fly with a competitor airline or if you're extra cautious, postpone your travel. To prevent this from happening, airports will practice physical distancing and rigorous sanitization. They will emphasize mask-wearing and conduct temperature checks at airport entrances. For some, traveling to certain parts of the world will also be restricted. For example, travelers from the US will not be permitted to enter Europe. Meanwhile, countries like Canada and Australia, not infested with the virus, will not face such travel restrictions.

We will continue to see fewer face-to-face purchases through brick-and-mortar stores with a shift towards increased e-commerce traffic. Unable to weather the economic storm, companies such as J. Crew, Pier 1, True Religion, and Virgin Australia have already filed for bankruptcy. Forever 21 may be forever gone. On the other hand, companies providing technologies to work remotely - such as Citrix and Zoom, pharmaceutical corporations, entertainment streaming vendors - such as Netflix and Hulu, and online marketplaces - such as Amazon, will continue to flourish.

As the current crisis calms, the citizens will seek new policies addressing pandemic preparedness from their elected officials. China will be scrutinized as other nations demand answers regarding the origin of the virus and will likely be penalized for its hiding of truth and disinformation tactics.

FUTURE THREATS

As one-third of humans worldwide faced some form of lockdown, the current pandemic will surely be remembered for centuries to come. World hunger, climate change, and pandemics are few of the future major threats to mankind.

As COVID-19 disrupts food supplies, the poor in developing countries are particularly vulnerable. Before the onset of the pandemic, 821 million people were estimated to be undernourished, as per the UN. Now, with the virus, developing countries face a double crisis – hunger and COVID-19. Countries like Ethiopia, Kenya, and Somalia are particularly susceptible due to recent droughts and harvest failures. During the Ebola crisis, food production in Africa dropped by 12%. Restrictions and market closures disrupted the flow of food. During the current pandemic, already weakened by hunger and compromised health, many in developing countries are particularly vulnerable to the novel coronavirus.

The UN World Food Programme estimates that the number of people starving worldwide could double due to the pandemic. That is a total of 265 million people - roughly the population of the UK, Germany, Italy, Spain, and Portugal combined, who could be pushed to the brink of starvation in 2020.[203] Some of the countries that witnessed the worst food crises in 2019 were the Democratic Republic of Congo, Yemen, Ethiopia, and Syria.[204] The UN's food relief agency officials stated that with enough funding, they could keep the supply chains open and position the food closer, thereby avoiding the famine.[205] In many parts of the world, the threat of hunger is more imminent than the virus. The virus amplifies famine by interrupting the transportation of food, disturbing agricultural production, and straining supply chains. Add insufficient medical care and poor infrastructure of these developing countries. If the virus spreads, this plight can rapidly evolve into a catastrophe. In countries including South Africa, Honduras, and India, frustrations from lockdowns and hunger have already begun to be channeled into protests and riots.[206,207,208]

The hard-learned lesson of how a problem in a different continent can quickly cost lives and jobs in one's home will be tested when humanity faces its unrivaled threat of climate change. Climate change, not unlike the viral pandemic, does not respect national borders. Undoubtedly, the effects of climate change will be felt worldwide. As the weather patterns change, sea levels rise, and climate-related disasters occur in increasing frequency and magnitude, climate scientists continue ringing the bell. Governments, industries, and global citizens must pay attention to these issues.

We have already started to witness many climate change-related calamities. From July 2019, Australian bushfires raged for more than 240 days following the hottest year on record. They have destroyed thousands of homes, killed more than a billion animals, cost the economy more than USD 3 billion, and burned 10.9 million hectares of land (approximately the size of Tennessee or Bulgaria).[209,210] South Asian floods resulted in more than 300,000 people being displaced and one-third of Bangladesh to be underwater.[211] The cyclones in March and April 2019 have killed more than 600 in Southern Africa and resulted in 160,000 people being displaced.[212]

Lockdowns, restrictions on travel, the size of a nation's arsenal, or advances in vaccination will not hinder climate change's ramifications. Once we're there, the time is up. All nations must work together to shrink their carbon footprints, incentivize renewable energy sources, stop deforestation, and reduce or eliminate meat from our diets.

In March 2020, the World Wildlife Fund surveyed 5,000 people in Hong Kong, Japan, Myanmar, Thailand, and Vietnam about their perceptions regarding the outbreak and their opinions on illegal and unregulated wildlife markets. Of the respondents, 79% felt that closure of unlawful and unregulated wildlife markets would prevent similar pandemics in the future. In light of COVID-19, 84% indicated that they would not purchase wildlife animal products in the future. Additionally, 93% stated that their governments would likely support the closure of such illegal and unregulated markets. Of the people who would continue to purchase wildlife products in the future, 41% would not buy such products from another source if the markets were to shut down. This survey indicated how effective potential wildlife market closures could be.[213]

The majority of emerging infectious diseases (60%) appear to be from animal origins (zoonotic).[214] Wet markets and industrial animal agriculture have been blamed in part for the increasing incidence of infectious diseases originating from animals. Crowding of factory farms with sick and stressed animals, along with unsanitary conditions, provides opportunities for viral mixing between animal hosts and the jump to the human population. These environments serve as a petri dish for new germs to emerge.

The original SARS outbreak of 2002 emerged from a wet market. In 1986, mad cow disease (bovine spongiform encephalopathy) resulted from cattle being fed infected meat. In 1996, as contaminated beef was consumed by humans, an outbreak of variant Creutzfeldt-Jakob disease (a fatal, dementia-like brain disorder) occurred. The 2009 H1N1 (Swine Flu) pandemic emerged from pigs in Mexico. If HIV originated from primates, as evidence suggests, the route of transmission was likely through infected simian blood from butchering of the animals for *bushmeat* consumption. Unfortunately, this practice continues to this day.[215] This maltreatment of animals is to be blamed, at least in part, for the rising infectious diseases. We then harm more animals in the lab during our pursuit of vaccinations and testing of new medications to combat diseases that occurred because of our maltreatment of animals to begin with. How about leaving animals alone in the first place? One could argue that what has been done in the past cannot be changed, and now we should do what we can to minimize human suffering. Fair, but we can improve our attitudes and behaviors now to reduce animal mistreatment, which is leading to our own peril. Animal consumption not only harms the animal and the person who consumes it, but it also threatens the wellbeing of others around the world and our future generations.[216]

Compared to all other mammals, bats have been recognized as harboring significantly higher proportions of viruses capable of infecting humans.[217] Rabies, SARS-CoV-1, MERS-CoV, SARS-CoV-2, Ebola, Nipah, and

Marburg viruses are some, from bat origin, known to have caused outbreaks of different magnitudes in humans. Bats have also been implicated behind the transmission of viruses threatening animal health. For instance, from 2016-2017, swine acute diarrhea syndrome coronavirus (SADS-CoV) was responsible for an outbreak in pigs, which killed more than 24,000 piglets in China.[218] Increasing spillover of diseases from host animals to humans and other animals has been apparent.

Human activities, by and large, are the primary drivers of the increase in zoonotic diseases. Operations, such as expanding agricultural practices, deforestation, and urbanization, which extend human interferences further into the uninhabited regions, are to be blamed.[219] One effective strategy appears to be to maintain humanity's distance from the wilderness.[220] Population growth, advancing human mobility, and the increased prevalence of chronic health conditions, in combination with growing global meat consumption giving rise to livestock production, are setting us up for future pandemics with concerning death tolls.[221]

What steps can we take to mitigate the effects of future pandemics? If pandemics will be recurring, as history and scientific evidence suggests, what about a pandemic response financial plan? Similar to plans that governments routinely conceive and practice for earthquakes, floods, or fires. Like the 2008 Financial Crisis, we witness government bailouts of large corporations who suffer financial losses due to this pandemic. Bailouts reduce the incentive for precautionary saving or pandemic insurance. Too good a fire department and people start storing gasoline in the basement.[222] The government and the private sector also need to devise a plan on how to keep public services (such as law enforcement and hospitals) and utilities (for example, electricity, water, Wi-Fi) operational if workers in those fields start falling ill.

In the future, when we reflect back to this period of COVID-19, the world will judge businesses based on how they treated their employees and customers. The governments will be judged based on their issued policies for the benefit of their citizens and how they collaborated with other countries for scarce resources. The nations of the world will be compared on how they conducted themselves, addressed the crisis, and ensured their healthcare facilities kept the number of deaths at minimum.

> *"The ultimate measure of a man is not where he stands in moments of comfort and convenience, but where he stands at times of challenge and controversy."*
>
> **Martin Luther King, Jr.**

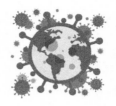

REFERENCES

1   *Naming the Coronavirus Disease (COVID-19) and the Virus That Causes It.* World Health Organization, www.who.int/emergencies/diseases/novel-coronavirus-2019/technical-guidance/naming-the-coronavirus-disease-(covid-2019)-and-the-virus-that-causes-it

2   Yan, Renhong, et al. "Structural Basis for the Recognition of SARS-CoV-2 by Full-Length Human ACE2." *Science*, vol. 367, no. 6485, 27 Mar. 2020, pp. 1444–1448, doi:10.1126/science. Ab 2762

3   Xiao, Kangpeng, et al. "Isolation and Characterization of 2019-NCoV-like Coronavirus from Malayan Pangolins." *BioRxiv*, 20 Feb. 2020, doi:10.1101/2020.02.17.951335

4   Xiao, Kangpeng, et al. "Isolation and Characterization of 2019-NCoV-like Coronavirus from Malayan Pangolins." *BioRxiv*, 20 Feb. 2020, doi:10.1101/2020.02.17.951335

5   Gandhi, Monica, et al. "Asymptomatic Transmission, the Achilles' Heel of Current Strategies to Control Covid-19." *New England Journal of Medicine*, 24 Apr. 2020, doi:10.1056/nejme2009758

6   Saito, Yasufumi, et al. "High-Speed Trains, International Flights: How the Coronavirus Spread." *The Wall Street Journal*, 5 Mar. 2020, www.wsj.com/graphics/how-the-coronavirus-spread/

7   Wilder-Smith, Annelies, et al. "Can We Contain the COVID-19 Outbreak with the Same Measures as for SARS?" *The Lancet Infectious Diseases*, 5 Mar. 2020, doi:10.1016/s1473-3099(20)30129-8

8   Keita, Sekou. "Air Passenger Mobility, Travel Restrictions, and the Transmission of the Covid-19 Pandemic between Countries." *COVID Economics*, no. 9, 24 Apr. 2020, pp. 77–96

9   Liu, Ying, et al. "The Reproductive Number of COVID-19 Is Higher Compared to SARS Coronavirus." *Journal of Travel Medicine*, vol. 27, no. 2, Mar. 2020

10   Moore, Kristine A., et al. *COVID-19: The CIDRAP Viewpoint. Part 1: The Future of the COVID-19 Pandemic: Lessons Learned from Pandemic Influenza.* 2020, *COVID-19: The CIDRAP Viewpoint. Part 1: The Future of the COVID-19 Pandemic: Lessons Learned from Pandemic Influenza,* www.cidrap.umn.edu/sites/default/files/public/downloads/cidrap-covid19-viewpoint-part1_0.pdf

11   *Coronavirus Disease 2019 (COVID-19) Situation Report – 73.* WHO, 2 Apr. 2020, www.who.int/docs/default-source/coronaviruse/situation-reports/20200402-sitrep-73-covid-19.pdf

12   Guo, Zhen-Dong, et al. "Aerosol and Surface Distribution of Severe Acute Respiratory Syndrome Coronavirus 2 in Hospital Wards, Wuhan, China, 2020." *Emerging Infectious Diseases*, vol. 26, no. 7, 2020, doi:10.3201/eid2607.200885

13   Doremalen, Neeltje Van, et al. "Aerosol and Surface Stability of SARS-CoV-2 as Compared with SARS-CoV-1." *New England Journal of Medicine*, vol. 382, no. 16, 16 Apr. 2020, pp. 1564–1567., doi:10.1056/nejmc2004973

14   Fu, Leiwen et al. "Clinical characteristics of coronavirus disease 2019 (COVID-19) in China: A systematic review and meta-analysis." *The Journal of infection*, S0163-4453(20)30170-5. 10 Apr. 2020, doi:10.1016/j.jinf.2020.03.041

15   Bialek, Stephanie, et al. "Severe Outcomes Among Patients with Coronavirus Disease 2019 (COVID-19) — United States, February 12–March 16, 2020." *MMWR. Morbidity and Mortality*

Weekly Report, vol. 69, no. 12, 27 Mar. 2020, pp. 343–346., doi:10.15585/mmwr.mm6912e2

16 Guan, Wei-Jie, et al. "Clinical Characteristics of Coronavirus Disease 2019 in China." *New England Journal of Medicine*, vol. 382, no. 18, 30 Apr. 2020, pp. 1708–1720., doi:10.1056/nejmoa2002032

17 Wang, Bolin, et al. "Does Comorbidity Increase the Risk of Patients with COVID-19: Evidence from Meta-Analysis." *Aging*, vol. 12, no. 7, 8 Apr. 2020, pp. 6049–6057., doi:10.18632/aging.103000

18 Mao, Ling, et al. "Neurologic Manifestations of Hospitalized Patients with Coronavirus Disease 2019 in Wuhan, China." *JAMA Neurology*, 10 Apr. 2020, doi:10.1001/jamaneurol.2020.1127

19 Zhou, Yunyun, et al. "Ocular Findings and Proportion with Conjunctival SARS-COV-2 in COVID-19 Patients." *Ophthalmology*, 21 Apr. 2020, doi:10.1016/j.ophtha.2020.04.028

20 Fu, Leiwen et al. "Clinical characteristics of coronavirus disease 2019 (COVID-19) in China: A systematic review and meta-analysis." *The Journal of infection*, S0163-4453(20)30170-5. 10 Apr. 2020, doi:10.1016/j.jinf.2020.03.041

21 Li, Bo, et al. "Prevalence and Impact of Cardiovascular Metabolic Diseases on COVID-19 in China." *Clinical Research in Cardiology*, vol. 109, no. 5, 11 Mar. 2020, pp. 531–538., doi:10.1007/s00392-020-01626-9

22 Wang, Dawei, et al. "Clinical Characteristics of 138 Hospitalized Patients With 2019 Novel Coronavirus–Infected Pneumonia in Wuhan, China." *Jama*, vol. 323, no. 11, 7 Feb. 2020, pp. 1061–1069., doi:10.1001/jama.2020.1585

23 Zhou, Fei, et al. "Clinical Course and Risk Factors for Mortality of Adult Inpatients with COVID-19 in Wuhan, China: A Retrospective Cohort Study." *The Lancet*, vol. 395, no. 10229, 28 Mar. 2020, pp. 1054–1062., doi:10.1016/s0140-6736(20)30566-3

24 Bansal, Manish. "Cardiovascular Disease and COVID-19." *Diabetes & Metabolic Syndrome: Clinical Research & Reviews*, vol. 14, no. 3, 25 Mar. 2020, pp. 247–250, doi:10.1016/j.dsx2020.03.013

25 Fu, Leiwen et al. "Clinical characteristics of coronavirus disease 2019 (COVID-19) in China: A systematic review and meta-analysis." *The Journal of infection*, S0163-4453(20)30170-5. 10 Apr. 2020, doi:10.1016/j.jinf.2020.03.041

26 Zhang, Jin-Jin, et al. "Clinical Characteristics of 140 Patients Infected with SARS-CoV-2 in Wuhan, China." *Allergy*, 19 Feb. 2020, doi:10.1111/all.14238

27 Recalcati, S. "Cutaneous Manifestations in COVID-19: A First Perspective." *Journal of the European Academy of Dermatology and Venereology*, 26 Mar. 2020, doi:10.1111/jdv.16387

28 Sachdeva, Muskaan, et al. "Cutaneous Manifestations of COVID-19: Report of Three Cases and a Review of Literature." *Journal of Dermatological Science*, 29 Apr. 2020, doi:10.1016/j.jdermsci.2020.04.011

29 Lai, Shengjie, et al. "Preliminary Risk Analysis of 2019 Novel Coronavirus Spread within and beyond China." *WorldPop*, 25 Jan. 2020, www.worldpop.org/events/china

30 Tognotti, Eugenia. "Lessons from the History of Quarantine, from Plague to Influenza A." *Emerging Infectious Diseases*, vol. 19, no. 2, Feb. 2013, pp. 254–259., doi:10.3201/eid1902.120312

31 Noel, Reginald A. *Race, Economics, And Social Status*. U.S. BUREAU OF LABOR STATISTICS, 2018, p. 2, *Race, Economics, And Social Status*

32 Rogers, Richard G., et al. *Living and Dying in the USA: Behavioral, Health, and Social Differentials of Adult Mortality*. Elsevier, 2007

33 Barnett, Karen, et al. "Epidemiology of Multimorbidity and Implications for Health Care, Research, and Medical Education: a Cross-Sectional Study." *The Lancet*, vol. 380, no. 9836, 10 May 2012, pp. 37–43., doi:10.1016/s0140-6736(12)60240-2

34 Moore, Kristine A., et al. *COVID-19: The CIDRAP Viewpoint. Part 1: The Future of the COVID-19 Pandemic: Lessons Learned from Pandemic Influenza*. 2020, *COVID-19: The CIDRAP Viewpoint. Part 1: The Future of the COVID-19 Pandemic: Lessons Learned from Pandemic Influenza*, www.cidrap.umn.edu/sites/

default/files/public/downloads/cidrap-covid19-viewpoint-part1_0.pdf

35 *1918 Pandemic Influenza: Three Waves.* Centers for Disease Control and Prevention, www.cdc.gov/flu/pandemic-resources/1918-pandemic-h1n1.html

36 Moore, Kristine A., et al. *COVID-19: The CIDRAP Viewpoint. Part 1: The Future of the COVID-19 Pandemic: Lessons Learned from Pandemic Influenza.* 2020, *COVID-19: The CIDRAP Viewpoint. Part 1: The Future of the COVID-19 Pandemic: Lessons Learned from Pandemic Influenza,* www.cidrap.umn.edu/sites/default/files/public/downloads/cidrap-covid19-viewpoint-part1_0.pdf

37 Lai, Shengjie, et al. "Effect of Non-Pharmaceutical Interventions for Containing the COVID-19 Outbreak in China." *MedRxiv,* 6 Mar. 2020, doi:10.1101/2020.03.03.20029843

38 Frost WH Statistics of influenza morbidity. Public Health Rep. 1920; 35:584–97 10.2307/4575511

39 Johnson NPAS, Mueller J. Updating the accounts: global mortality of the 1918–1920 "Spanish" influenza pandemic. Bull Hist Med. 2002; 76:105–115

40 Frost WH Statistics of influenza morbidity. Public Health Rep. 1920; 35:584–97 10.2307/4575511

41 Humphries, Mark Osborne. "Paths of Infection: The First World War and the Origins of the 1918 Influenza Pandemic." *War in History,* vol. 21, no. 1, 8 Jan. 2014, pp. 55–81., doi:10.1177/0968344513504525

42 Saunders-Hastings, Patrick, and Daniel Krewski. "Reviewing the History of Pandemic Influenza: Understanding Patterns of Emergence and Transmission." *Pathogens,* vol. 5, no. 4, 6 Dec. 2016, doi:10.3390/pathogens5040066

43 Moore, Kristine A., et al. *COVID-19: The CIDRAP Viewpoint. Part 1: The Future of the COVID-19 Pandemic: Lessons Learned from Pandemic Influenza.* 2020, *COVID-19: The CIDRAP Viewpoint. Part 1: The Future of the COVID-19 Pandemic: Lessons Learned from Pandemic Influenza,* www.cidrap.umn.edu/sites/default/files/public/downloads/cidrap-covid19-viewpoint-part1_0.pdf

44   Biggerstaff, M., Cauchemez, S., Reed, C. et al. Estimates of the reproduction number for seasonal, pandemic, and zoonotic influenza: a systematic review of the literature. *BMC Infect Dis* 14, 480 (2014). https://doi.org/10.1186/1471-2334-14-480

45   Cécile Viboud, Lone Simonsen, Rodrigo Fuentes, Jose Flores, Mark A. Miller, Gerardo Chowell, Global Mortality Impact of the 1957–1959 Influenza Pandemic, *The Journal of Infectious Diseases*, Volume 213, Issue 5, 1 March 2016, Pages 738–745, https://doi.org/10.1093/infdis/jiv534

46   Henderson, D. A., et al. "Public Health and Medical Responses to the 1957-58 Influenza Pandemic." *Biosecurity and Bioterrorism: Biodefense Strategy, Practice, and Science*, vol. 7, no. 3, 2009, pp. 265–273., doi:10.1089/bsp.2009.0729

47   Saunders-Hastings, Patrick, and Daniel Krewski. "Reviewing the History of Pandemic Influenza: Understanding Patterns of Emergence and Transmission." *Pathogens*, vol. 5, no. 4, 6 Dec. 2016, doi:10.3390/pathogens5040066

48   Viboud, Cécile, et al. "Multinational Impact of the 1968 Hong Kong Influenza Pandemic: Evidence for a Smoldering Pandemic." *The Journal of Infectious Diseases*, vol. 192, no. 2, 15 July 2005, pp. 233–248., doi:10.1086/431150

49   *1968 Pandemic (H3N2 Virus).* Centers for Disease Control and Prevention, www.cdc.gov/flu/pandemic-resources/1968-pandemic.html

50   Saunders-Hastings, Patrick, and Daniel Krewski. "Reviewing the History of Pandemic Influenza: Understanding Patterns of Emergence and Transmission." *Pathogens*, vol. 5, no. 4, 6 Dec. 2016, doi:10.3390/pathogens5040066

51   Jones, Kate E., et al. "Global Trends in Emerging Infectious Diseases." *Nature*, vol. 451, no. 7181, 21 Feb. 2008, pp. 990–993., doi:10.1038/nature06536

52   Lessler, Justin, et al. "Outbreak of 2009 Pandemic Influenza A (H1N1) at a New York City School: NEJM." *New England Journal of Medicine*, 13 Apr. 2020, www.nejm.org/doi/full/10.1056/NEJMoa0906089

53 Saunders-Hastings, Patrick, and Daniel Krewski. "Reviewing the History of Pandemic Influenza: Understanding Patterns of Emergence and Transmission." *Pathogens*, vol. 5, no. 4, 6 Dec. 2016, doi:10.3390/pathogens5040066

54 DEPARTMENT OF COMMUNICABLE DISEASE SURVEILLANCE AND RESPONSE. *Consensus Document on the Epidemiology of Severe Acute Respiratory Syndrome (SARS)*. WHO, 2003, p. 8 www.who.int/csr/sars/en/WHOconsensus.pdf

55 DEPARTMENT OF COMMUNICABLE DISEASE SURVEILLANCE AND RESPONSE. *Consensus Document on the Epidemiology of Severe Acute Respiratory Syndrome (SARS)*. WHO, 2003, p. 27 www.who.int/csr/sars/en/WHOconsensus.pdf

56 DEPARTMENT OF COMMUNICABLE DISEASE SURVEILLANCE AND RESPONSE. *Consensus Document on the Epidemiology of Severe Acute Respiratory Syndrome (SARS)*. WHO, 2003, p. 10 www.who.int/csr/sars/en/WHOconsensus.pdf

57 Chang, Hyuk-Jun. "Estimation of Basic Reproduction Number of the Middle East Respiratory Syndrome Coronavirus (MERS-CoV) during the Outbreak in South Korea, 2015." *BioMedical Engineering OnLine*, vol. 16, 13 June 2017, doi:10.1186/s12938-017-0370-7

58 *MERS Situation Update*. WHO, 2019, applications.emro.who.int/docs/EMRPUB-CSR-241-2019-EN.pdf?ua=1&ua=1&ua=1

59 MERS-CoV Global Summary and Assessment of Risk, July 2019 (WHO/MERS/RA/19.1). Geneva, Switzerland: World Health Organization; 2019. Licence: CC BY-NC-SA 3.0 IGO

60 Rohan, Hana, and Gillian Mckay. "The Ebola Outbreak in the Democratic Republic of the Congo: Why There Is No 'Silver Bullet.'" *Nature Immunology*, 21 Apr. 2020, doi:10.1038/s41590-020-0675-8

61 Rohan, Hana, and Gillian Mckay. "The Ebola Outbreak in the Democratic Republic of the Congo: Why There Is No 'Silver Bullet.'" *Nature Immunology*, 21 Apr. 2020, doi:10.1038/s41590-020-0675-8

62 Wells, Chad R., et al. "The Exacerbation of Ebola Outbreaks by Conflict in the Democratic Republic of the Congo." *Proceedings*

of the National Academy of Sciences, vol. 116, no. 48, 21 Oct. 2019, pp. 24366–24372., doi:10.1073/pnas.1913980116

63 *Ebola Virus Disease*. World Health Organization, 10 Feb. 2020, www.who.int/news-room/fact-sheets/detail/ebola-virus-disease

64 Rojek, A.m., et al. "A Systematic Review and Meta-Analysis of Patient Data from the West Africa (2013–16) Ebola Virus Disease Epidemic." *Clinical Microbiology and Infection*, vol. 25, no. 11, 5 July 2019, pp. 1307–1314., doi:10.1016/j.cmi.2019.06.032

65 *Major Milestone for WHO-Supported Ebola Vaccine*. World Health Organization, www.who.int/news-room/detail/18-10-2019-major-milestone-for-who-supported-ebola-vaccine

66 "Influenza (Seasonal)." *Influenza (Seasonal)*, World Health Organization, 6 Nov. 2018, www.who.int/en/news-room/fact-sheets/detail/influenza-(seasonal).

67 Lessler, Justin, et al. "Incubation Periods of Acute Respiratory Viral Infections: A Systematic Review." *The Lancet Infectious Diseases*, vol. 9, no. 5, May 2009, pp. 291–300., doi:10.1016/s1473-3099(09)70069-6

68 Biggerstaff, M., Cauchemez, S., Reed, C. *et al.* Estimates of the reproduction number for seasonal, pandemic, and zoonotic influenza: a systematic review of the literature. *BMC Infect Dis* 14, 480 (2014). https://doi.org/10.1186/1471-2334-14-480

69 Moghadami, Mohsen. "A Narrative Review of Influenza: A Seasonal and Pandemic Disease." *Iranian journal of medical sciences* vol. 42,1 (2017): 2-13

70 "Estimates of Influenza Vaccination Coverage among Adults-United States, 2017–18 Flu Season." *Centers for Disease Control and Prevention*, Centers for Disease Control and Prevention, 5 Nov. 2018, www.cdc.gov/flu/fluvaxview/coverage-1718estimates.htm.

71 Canada, Public Health Agency of. "Government of Canada." *Canada.ca*, 21 Mar. 2019, www.canada.ca/en/public-health/services/publications/healthy-living/2017-2018-seasonal-influenza-flu-vaccine-coverage-survey-results.html.

72   "44% Of Elderly People Vaccinated against Influenza." *44% Of Elderly People Vaccinated against Influenza - Product - Eurostat*, ec.europa.eu/eurostat/web/products-eurostat-news/-/DDN-20191209-2.

73   Hu, Ben, et al. "Discovery of a Rich Gene Pool of Bat SARS-Related Coronaviruses Provides New Insights into the Origin of SARS Coronavirus." *PLOS Pathogens*, vol. 13, no. 11, e1006698. 30 Nov. 2017. doi:10.1371/journal.ppat 1006698

74   Ge, Xing-Yi, et al. "Isolation and Characterization of a Bat SARS-like Coronavirus That Uses the ACE2 Receptor." *Nature*, vol. 503, no. 7477, 30 Oct. 2013, pp. 535–538., doi:10.1038/nature12711

75   Wang, Ning, et al. "Serological Evidence of Bat SARS-Related Coronavirus Infection in Humans, China." *Virologica Sinica*, vol. 33, 2 Mar. 2018, pp. 104–107., doi:10.1007/s12250-018-0012-7

76   Menachery, Vineet D, et al. "A SARS-like Cluster of Circulating Bat Coronaviruses Shows Potential for Human Emergence." *Nature Medicine*, vol. 21, 9 Nov. 2015, pp. 1508–1513., doi:10.1038/nm.3985

77   Chowell, G. et al. Transmission characteristics of MERS and SARS in the healthcare setting: a comparative study. *BMC Med.* 13, 210 (2015). An analysis of the predominant role for nosocomial transmission in the epidemiology of both SARS and MERS

78   Hunter, J. C. et al. Transmission of Middle East respiratory syndrome coronavirus infections in healthcare settings, Abu Dhabi. *Emerg. Infect. Dis.* 22, 647–656 (2016)

79   Lee, Nelson, and Joseph J.Y. Sung. "Nosocomial Transmission of SARS." *Current Infectious Disease Reports*, vol. 5, no. 6, 2003, pp. 473–476., doi:10.1007/s11908-003-0089-4

80   Anderson, R. M. et al. Epidemiology, transmission dynamics and control of SARS: the 2002–2003 epidemic. *Philos. Trans. R. Soc. Lond. B. Biol. Sci.* 359, 1091–1105 (2004)

81   Crowling, B. J. et al. Preliminary epidemiological assessment of MERS-CoV outbreak in South Korea, May to June 2015. *Euro Surveill.* 20, 7–13 (2015)

82   Chowell, G. et al. Transmission characteristics of MERS and SARS in the healthcare setting: a comparative study. *BMC Med.* 13, 210 (2015). An analysis of the predominant role for nosocomial transmission in the epidemiology of both SARS and MERS

83   Hunter, J. C. et al. Transmission of Middle East respiratory syndrome coronavirus infections in healthcare settings, Abu Dhabi. *Emerg. Infect. Dis.* 22, 647–656 (2016)

84   Wang, Dawei, et al. "Clinical Characteristics of 138 Hospitalized Patients With 2019 Novel Coronavirus–Infected Pneumonia in Wuhan, China." *JAMA*, vol. 323, no. 11, 7 Feb. 2020, pp. 1061–1069., doi:10.1001/jama.2020.1585

85   Knobler, Stacey, et al. *Learning from SARS Preparing for the next Disease Outbreak: Workshop Summary.* National Academies Press, 2004

86   Menachery, Vineet D, et al. "A SARS-like Cluster of Circulating Bat Coronaviruses Shows Potential for Human Emergence." *Nature Medicine*, vol. 21, 9 Nov. 2015, pp. 1508–1513., doi:10.1038/nm.3985

87   Menachery, Vineet D., et al. "SARS-like WIV1-CoV Poised for Human Emergence." *Proceedings of the National Academy of Sciences*, vol. 113, no. 11, 14 Mar. 2016, pp. 3048–3053., doi:10.1073/pnas.1517719113

88   "Our Data." *Get Us PPE*, getusppe.org/data

89   Fink, S. Worst-case estimates for U.S. coronavirus deaths. New York Times. March 18, 2020 (https://www.nytimes.com/2020/03/13/us/coronavirus-deaths-estimate.html)

90   Rubinson, Lewis, et al. "Mechanical Ventilators in US Acute Care Hospitals." *Disaster Medicine and Public Health Preparedness*, U.S. National Library of Medicine, Oct. 2010, www.ncbi.nlm.nih.gov/pubmed/21149215

91   Rubinson, Lewis, et al. "Mechanical Ventilators in US Acute Care Hospitals." *Disaster Medicine and Public Health Preparedness*, U.S. National Library of Medicine, Oct. 2010, www.ncbi.nlm.nih.gov/pubmed/21149215

92   Zhou, Fei, et al. *Clinical Course and Risk Factors for Mortality of Adult Inpatients with COVID-19 in Wuhan, China: a Retrospective Cohort Study.* The Lancet, 11 Mar. 2020, www.thelancet.com/journals/lancet/article/PIIS0140-6736(20)30566-3/fulltext

93   Richardson, Safiya, et al. "Presenting Characteristics, Comorbidities, and Outcomes Among 5700 Patients Hospitalized With COVID-19 in the New York City Area." *JAMA*, 22 Apr. 2020, doi:10.1001/jama.2020.6775

94   Ajao, A. Nystrom SV, Koonin LM, et al. Assessing the capacity of the US health care system to use additional mechanical ventilators during a large-scale public health emergency. Disaster Med Public Health Prep 2015;9(6):634-641. doi:10.1017/dmp.2015.105

95   *Ethical Considerations for Decision Regarding Allocation of Mechanical Ventilators during a Severe Influenza Pandemic or Other Public Health Emergency.* CDC.gov, 1 July 2011, www.cdc.gov/od/science/integrity/phethics/docs/Vent_Document_Final_Version.pdf

96   Burkle FM, Jr. Mass casualty management of a large-scale bioterrorist event: An epidemiological approach that shapes triage decisions. Emerg Med Clin North Am 2002;20:409-436

97   *Ethical Considerations for Decision Regarding Allocation of Mechanical Ventilators during a Severe Influenza Pandemic or Other Public Health Emergency.* CDC.gov, 1 July 2011, www.cdc.gov/od/science/integrity/phethics/docs/Vent_Document_Final_Version.pdf

98   Lo, B. White, DB. Intensive care unit triage during an influenza pandemic: The need for specific clinical guidelines. In Lemon SM, Hamburg MA, Sparling F, Choffnes ER, Mack A (Eds). Ethical and Legal Considerations in Mitigating Pandemic Disease. Washington, D.C.: National Academies Press; 2007, pp. 192-197

99   *Ethical Considerations for Decision Regarding Allocation of Mechanical Ventilators during a Severe Influenza Pandemic or Other Public Health Emergency.* CDC.gov, 1 July 2011, www.cdc.gov/od/science/integrity/phethics/docs/Vent_Document_Final_Version.pdf

100 Zundel K. M. (1996). Telemedicine: history, applications, and impact on librarianship. *Bulletin of the Medical Library Association*, *84*(1), 71–79

101 Armfield NR, Bradford M, Bradford NK. The clinical use of Skype—for which patients, with which problems and in which settings? A snapshot review of the literature. *Int J Med Inform*2015;84:737-42. doi:10.1016/j.ijmedinf.2015.06.006 pmid:26183642

102 Backhaus A, Agha Z, Maglione ML, et al. Videoconferencing psychotherapy: a systematic review. *Psychol Serv*2012;9:111-31. doi:10.1037/a0027924 pmid:22662727

103 World Health Organization Statement on the 1st meeting of the IHR Emergency Committee on the 2014 Ebola outbreak in West Africa (2014) http://www.who.int/mediacentre/news/statements/2014/ebola-20140808/en/

104 Busting the myths about Ebola is crucial to stop the transmission of the disease in Guinea (2014) http://www.who.int/features/2014/ebola-myths/en/

105 Gravenstein, JS, et al. "Laser Mediated Telemedicine in Anesthesia" *LWW*, Anesthesia & Analgesia, July/Aug 1974

106 Telemedicine in critical care: An experiment in health care delivery. Grundy, Betty L. et al. Journal of the American College of Emergency Physicians, Volume 6, Issue 10, 439 – 444

107 Lilly, Craig M., et al. "Critical Care Telemedicine." *Critical Care Medicine*, vol. 42, no. 11, Nov. 2014, pp. 2429–2436., doi:10.1097/ccm.0000000000000539.

108 Zundel, K. M. (1996). Telemedicine: history, applications, and impact on librarianship. *Bulletin of the Medical Library Association*, *84*(1), 71–79

109 Caldarola, Pasquale, et al. "ANMCO/SIT Consensus Document: Telemedicine for Cardiovascular Emergency Networks." *European Heart Journal Supplements*, vol. 19, no. suppl_D, 2017, pp. D229–D243., doi:10.1093/eurheartj/sux028

110 Zollo, S, Kienzle M, Henshaw Z, Crist L, Wakefield D. Tele-education in a telemedicine environment: implications for rural health care and academic medical centers. J Med Syst. 1999;23(2):107–22

111 Sadique, Md Z et al. "Estimating the costs of school closure for mitigating an influenza pandemic." *BMC public health* vol. 8 135. 24 Apr. 2008, doi:10.1186/1471-2458-8-135

112 Lempel, Howard et al. "Economic cost and health care workforce effects of school closures in the U.S." *PLoS currents* vol. 1 RRN1051. 5 Oct. 2009, doi:10.1371/currents.rrn1051

113 Patrick GT Walker, Charles Whittaker, Oliver Watson et al. The Global Impact of COVID-19 and Strategies for Mitigation and Suppression. Imperial College London (2020), doi: https://doi.org/10.25561/77735

114 White, KA. Pittsburgh in the Great Epidemic of 1918. W Pa Hist Mag. 1985;68:221–242

115 White, KA. Pittsburgh in the Great Epidemic of 1918. W Pa Hist Mag. 1985;68:221–242

116 Bootsma, Martin C. J., and Neil M. Ferguson. "The Effect of Public Health Measures on the 1918 Influenza Pandemic in U.S. Cities." *Proceedings of the National Academy of Sciences*, vol. 104, no. 18, 2007, pp. 7588–7593., doi:10.1073/pnas.0611071104

117 Hatchett, Richard J., et al. "Public Health Interventions and Epidemic Intensity during the 1918 Influenza Pandemic." *Proceedings of the National Academy of Sciences*, vol. 104, no. 18, 6 Apr. 2007, pp. 7582–7587., doi:10.1073/pnas.0610941104

118 Neil M Ferguson, Daniel Laydon, Gemma Nedjati-Gilani et al. Impact of non-pharmaceutical interventions (NPIs) to reduce COVID-19 mortality and healthcare demand. Imperial College London (16-03-2020), doi: https://doi.org/10.25561/77482

119 Neil M Ferguson, Daniel Laydon, Gemma Nedjati-Gilani et al. Impact of non-pharmaceutical interventions (NPIs) to reduce COVID-19 mortality and healthcare demand. Imperial College London (16-03-2020), doi: https://doi.org/10.25561/77482

120 "UNESCO Rallies International Organizations, Civil Society and Private Sector Partners in a Broad Coalition to Ensure #LearningNeverStops." *UNESCO*, 26 Mar. 2020, en.unesco.

org/news/unesco-rallies-international-organizations-civil-soci-ety-and-private-sector-partners-broad

121 "Child Nutrition Tables." *USDA Food and Nutrition Service*, www.fns.usda.gov/pd/child-nutrition-tables

122 Nafisah, Sharafaldeen Bin, et al. "School Closure during Novel Influenza: A Systematic Review." *Journal of Infection and Public Health*, vol. 11, no. 5, 2018, pp. 657–661., doi:10.1016/j.jiph.2018.01.003

123 Fung, Isaac Chun-Hai, et al. "Modeling the Effect of School Closures in a Pandemic Scenario: Exploring Two Different Contact Matrices." *Clinical Infectious Diseases*, vol. 60, no. suppl_1, 10 Apr. 2015, pp. S58–S63., doi:10.1093/cid/civ086

124 Gollier, Christian, and Oliver Gossner. "Group Testing against Covid-19." *Covid Economics*, no. 2, 8 Apr. 2020, pp. 32–42., cepr.org/sites/default/files/news/CovidEconomics2.pdf

125 Gollier, Christian, and Oliver Gossner. "Group Testing against Covid-19." *Covid Economics*, no. 2, 8 Apr. 2020, pp. 32–42., cepr.org/sites/default/files/news/CovidEconomics2.pdf

126 Okba, Nisreen M.a., et al. "Severe Acute Respiratory Syndrome Coronavirus 2–Specific Antibody Responses in Coronavirus Disease 2019 Patients." *Emerging Infectious Diseases*, vol. 26, no. 7, 8 Apr. 2020, doi:10.3201/eid2607.200841

127 "Roche's COVID-19 Antibody Test Receives FDA Emergency Use Authorization and Is Available in Markets Accepting the CE Mark." *Roche*, www.roche.com/media/releases/med-cor-2020-05-03.htm

128 Chan. *The Power of Vaccines: Still Not Fully Utilized*. World Health Organization, www.who.int/publications/10-year-re-view/vaccines/en

129 Pronker, Esther S., et al. "Risk in Vaccine Research and Development Quantified." *PLoS ONE*, vol. 8, no. 3, 20 Mar. 2013, doi:10.1371/journal.pone.0057755

130 "Vaccine Types." *Vaccines.gov*, U.S. Department of Health & Human Services, www.vaccines.gov/basics/types

131 *Principles of Vaccination*. CDC.gov, www.cdc.gov/vaccines/pubs/pinkbook/downloads/prinvac.pdf

132 Takano, Tomomi, et al. "Pathogenesis of Oral Type I Feline Infectious Peritonitis Virus (FIPV) Infection: Antibody-Dependent Enhancement Infection of Cats with Type I FIPV via the
Oral Route." *Journal of Veterinary Medical Science*, vol. 81, no.
6, 2019, pp. 911–915., doi:10.1292/jvms.18-0702

133 Khandia, Rekha, et al. "Modulation of Dengue/Zika Virus
Pathogenicity by Antibody-Dependent Enhancement and Strategies to Protect Against Enhancement in Zika Virus Infection."
Frontiers in Immunology, vol. 9, 23 Apr. 2018, pp. 313–324.,
doi:10.3389/fimmu.2018.00597

134 Hatchett, Richard J., et al. "Public Health Interventions and
Epidemic Intensity during the 1918 Influenza Pandemic." *Pro-
ceedings of the National Academy of Sciences*, vol. 104, no. 18, 6
Apr. 2007, pp. 7582–7587., doi:10.1073/pnas.0610941104

135 Pronker, Esther S., et al. "Risk in Vaccine Research and Development Quantified." *PLoS ONE*, vol. 8, no. 3, 20 Mar. 2013,
doi:10.1371/journal.pone.0057755

136 Le, Tung Thanh, et al. "The COVID-19 Vaccine Development
Landscape." *Nature Reviews Drug Discovery*, vol. 19, no. 5, 9
Apr. 2020, pp. 305–306., doi:10.1038/d41573-020-00073-5

137 HHS (Department of Health and Human Services). Appendix
D in Pandemic Influenza Plan. Washington, DC: Department
of Health and Human Services; 2005. [accessed December 27,
2006].

138 "Business Cycle Dating Committee, National Bureau of Economic Research." *National Bureau of Economic Research*, 20 Sept.
2010, www.nber.org/cycles/sept2010.html

139 Baldwin, Richard, and Beatrice Weder di Mauro. "Introduction"
Economics in the Time of Covid-19, Center for Economic Policy
Research, 2020, p. 2

140 Desjardins, Jeff. "The $80 Trillion World Economy in One
Chart." *Visual Capitalist*, 10 Oct. 2018, www.visualcapitalist.
com/80-trillion-world-economy-one-chart/

141 *The New Coronavirus Could Have a Lasting Impact on Global Supply Chains*. The Economist, 15 Feb.
2020, www.economist.com/international/2020/02/15/

the-new-coronavirus-could-have-a-lasting-impact-on-global-supply-chains

142 "An Unprecedented Plunge in Oil Demand Will Turn the Industry Upside Down." *The Economist*, The Economist Newspaper, 8 Apr. 2020, www.economist.com/briefing/2020/04/08/an-unprecedented-plunge-in-oil-demand-will-turn-the-industry-upside-down

143 https://www.bloomberg.com/news/articles/2020-04-08/world-economy-faces-5-trillion-hit-that-is-like-losing-japan?srnd=premium-europe

144 "THE EMPLOYMENT SITUATION — APRIL 2020." *Bureau of Labor Statistics*, 8 May 2020, www.bls.gov/news.release/pdf/empsit.pdf

145 Jackson, James, et al. *Global Economic Effects of COVID-19*. Congressional Research Service, 2020, p. 2, *Global Economic Effects of COVID-19*

146 Lebergott, Stanley. *Labor Force, Employment, and Unemployment, 1929-39: Estimating Methods*. www.bls.gov/opub/mlr/1948/article/pdf/labor-force-employment-and-unemployment-1929-39-estimating-methods.pdf

147 "The Recession of 2007–2009." *BLS Spotlight on Statistics*, Feb. 2012, www.bls.gov/spotlight/2012/recession/pdf/recession_bls_spotlight.pdf

148 "Unemployment Insurance Weekly Claims." *News Release*, US Department of Labor, 16 Apr. 2020, www.dol.gov/ui/data.pdf

149 Reinicke, Carmen. *US Weekly Jobless Claims Hit 5.2 Million, Wiping out All Jobs Created since the Great Recession in Just 4 Weeks*. Business Insider, 16 Apr. 2020, www.businessinsider.com/us-weekly-jobless-claims-labor-market-unemployment-filings-recession-coronavirus-2020-4

150 https://www.bloomberg.com/news/articles/2020-03-22/fed-s-bullard-says-u-s-jobless-rate-may-soar-to-30-in-2q?mod=article_inline

151 Pew Research Center, April 2020, "About Half of Lower-Income Americans Report Household Job or Wage Loss Due to COVID-19

152 "US Small Business Owners Face Great Uncertainty; Over Half Say They Cannot Operate Beyond Three Months." *10,000 Small Businesses*, 19 Mar. 2020, www.goldmansachs.com/citizenship/10000-small-businesses/US/no-time-to-waste/.

153 *ADVANCE MONTHLY SALES FOR RETAIL AND FOOD SERVICES, MARCH 2020*. U.S. Census Bureau, 15 Apr. 2020, www.census.gov/retail/marts/www/marts_current.pdf

154 "INDUSTRIAL PRODUCTION AND CAPACITY UTILIZATION." *FEDERAL RESERVE Statistical Release*, Federal Reserve, 15 Apr. 2020, www.federalreserve.gov/releases/g17/current/g17.pdf

155 Reinicke, Carmen. *US Factory Output Falls the Most since 1946 as the Coronavirus Lockdown Halts Activity*. Business Insider, 15 Apr. 2020, www.businessinsider.com/us-factory-output-march-declines-most-since-coronavirus-halt-industrial-2020-4

156 "China Percent of World GDP - Data, Chart." *TheGlobalEconomy.com*, www.theglobaleconomy.com/China/gdp_share/.

157 Baldwin, Richard, and Beatrice Weder di Mauro. "Trade and travel in the time of epidemics" *Economics in the Time of Covid-19*, Center for Economic Policy Research, 2020, p. 94

158 "Industry Losses to Top $84 Billion in 2020." *IATA*, 9 July 2020, www.iata.org/en/pressroom/pr/2020-06-09-01/.

159 "Industry Losses to Top $84 Billion in 2020." *IATA*, 9 July 2020, www.iata.org/en/pressroom/pr/2020-06-09-01/.

160 Rodriguez, Ashley. "How Netflix Usage Changed in 14 Countries in March, According to Exclusive App-Tracking Data." *Business Insider*, Business Insider, 15 Apr. 2020, www.businessinsider.com/netflix-app-data-suggests-countries-where-netflix-users-increased-q1-2020-4

161 Yuan, Eric S. "A Message to Our Users." *Zoom Blog*, 1 Apr. 2020, blog.zoom.us/wordpress/2020/04/01/a-message-to-our-users/.

162 Adrjan Pawel, and Reamonn Lydon. Central Bank of Ireland, 2020, pp. 2–2, *Covid-19 and the Global Labour Market: Impact on Job Postings*

163 Battersby, Bryn, et al. "Tracking the $9 Trillion Global Fiscal Support to Fight COVID-19." *IMF Blog*, 20 May 2020, blogs.

imf.org/2020/05/20/tracking-the-9-trillion-global-fiscal-support-to-fight-covid-19

164 Glover, Andrew, et al. "Health versus Wealth: On the Distributional Effects of Controlling a Pandemic." *Center for Economic Policy Research*, 16 Apr. 2020, no. 6, pp. 22–63

165 Melaine, Gbêtondji, and Armel Nonvide. "Short-Term Impact of COVID-19 on Poverty in Africa." *Covid Economics*, no. 15, 7 May 2020, pp. 184–195

166 Adams-Prassl, Abigail, et al. "The Large and Unequal Impact of COVID-19 on Workers." *The Large and Unequal Impact of COVID-19 on Workers | VOX, CEPR Policy Portal*, VoxEu, 8 Apr. 2020, voxeu.org/article/large-and-unequal-impact-covid-19-workers

167 Zhang, Stephen X et al. "Unprecedented disruption of lives and work: Health, distress and life satisfaction of working adults in China one month into the COVID-19 outbreak." *Psychiatry research*, vol. 288 112958. 4 Apr. 2020, doi:10.1016/j.psychres.2020.112958

168 Adams-Prassl, Abigail, et al. "The Large and Unequal Impact of COVID-19 on Workers." *The Large and Unequal Impact of COVID-19 on Workers | VOX, CEPR Policy Portal*, VoxEu, 8 Apr. 2020, voxeu.org/article/large-and-unequal-impact-covid-19-workers

169 Dingel, Jonathan, and Brent Neiman. "How Many Jobs Can Be Done from Home?" *Covid Economics*, CEPR Press, 3 Apr. 2020, cepr.org/sites/default/files/news/CovidEcon1%20final.pdf

170 Saltiel, Fernando. "Who Can Work from Home in Developing Countries?" *Covid Economics*, no. 6, 17 Apr. 2020, pp. 104–118., cepr.org/sites/default/files/news/CovidEconomics6.pdf

171 Wang, Dawei, et al. "Clinical Characteristics of 138 Hospitalized Patients With 2019 Novel Coronavirus–Infected Pneumonia in Wuhan, China." *Jama*, vol. 323, no. 11, 7 Feb. 2020, pp. 1061–1069., doi:10.1001/jama.2020.1585

172 Gottlieb, Charles, et al. "Working from Home across Countries." *Covid Economics*, no. 8, 22 Apr 2020, pp 71–91

173 Baker, Scott R. "The Unprecedented Stock Market Reaction to Covid-19." *CEPR Press*, no. 1, 3 Apr. 2020, pp. 33–40

174 Schoenfeld, Jordan. "The Invisible Risk: Pandemics and the Financial Markets." *Covid Economics*, no. 6, 17 Apr. 2020, pp. 119–136., cepr.org/sites/default/files/news/CovidEconomics6.pdf

175 Koren, Miklos, and Rita Peto. "Business Disruptions from Social Distancing." *Covid Economics*, no. 2, 8 Apr. 2020, pp. 13–28., cepr.org/sites/default/files/news/CovidEconomics2.pdf

176 Phillips, Tom, et al. "Covid-19: How World Leaders Responded to the Crisis." *The Guardian*, Guardian News and Media, 12 Apr. 2020, www.theguardian.com/world/2020/apr/12/covid-19-how-world-leaders-responded-to-the-crisis

177 Marin, Cecile. "Europe Versus Coronavirus - Putting the Danish Model to the Test." *Institut Montaigne*, Institut Montaigne, 12 May 2020, www.institutmontaigne.org/en/blog/europe-versus-coronavirus-putting-danish-model-test

178 "How the Coronavirus Outbreak Is Impacting Public Opinion." *Morning Consult*, morningconsult.com/form/coronavirus-outbreak-tracker/.

179 Murray, Shoon. "The 'Rally-'Round-the-Flag' Phenomenon and the Diversionary Use of Force." *Oxford Research Encyclopedia of Politics*, June 2017, doi:10.1093/acrefore/9780190228637.013.518

180 Hetherington, Marc J., and Michael Nelson. "Anatomy of a Rally Effect: George W. Bush and the War on Terrorism." *Political Science and Politics*, vol. 36, no. 01, 25 Apr. 2017, pp. 37–42., doi:10.1017/s1049096503001665

181 Manhire, Toby. "Almost 90% of New Zealanders Back Ardern Government on Covid-19 – Poll." *The Spinoff*, The Spinoff, 8 Apr. 2020, thespinoff.co.nz/politics/08-04-2020/almost-90-of-new-zealanders-back-ardern-government-on-covid-19-poll

182 Strongman, Susan. *Covid-19 Pandemic Timeline*, shorthand.radionz.co.nz/coronavirus-timeline/#section-nNAZ2NMUhk

183 *Protection Racket*. The Economist Newspaper, 23 Apr. 2020, www.economist.com/international/2020/04/23/would-be-autocrats-are-using-covid-19-as-an-excuse-to-grab-more-power

184   *A Pandemic of Power Grabs.* The Economist Newspaper, 23 Apr. 2020, www.economist.com/leaders/2020/04/23/autocrats-see-opportunity-in-disaster

185   Cupolo, Diego. "Turkish Political Prisoners Left out of Plan to Reduce Jail Population." *Al-Monitor,* 1 Apr. 2020, www.al-monitor.com/pulse/originals/2020/04/turkey-political-prisoners-remain-jail-pandemic.html

186   *American Wars.* Department of Veterans Affairs, Nov. 2019 https://www.va.gov/opa/publications/factsheets/fs_americas_wars.pdf

187   *Opening Up America Again.* The White House, www.whitehouse.gov/openingamerica/#criteria

188   Cohen, John. "Axios: SurveyMonkey Poll: Perceptions of Coronavirus." *SurveyMonkey,* www.surveymonkey.com/curiosity/axios-coronavirus-perception/?mod=article_inline

189   *Quinnipiac University Poll,* 9 Mar. 2020, poll.qu.edu/national/release-detail?ReleaseID=3657#.XmaSrM7okEs.twitter

190   Lash, Nathaniel, and Gus Wezerek. *Why Georgia Isn't Ready to Reopen, in Charts.* The New York Times, 24 Apr. 2020, www.nytimes.com/interactive/2020/04/24/opinion/coronavirus-covid-19-georgia-reopen.html

191   *To Live and Die in Dixie.* The Economist Newspaper, 21 Apr. 2020, www.economist.com/united-states/2020/04/21/covid-19-is-spreading-to-americas-south-with-unnerving-speed

192   Okoro, Catherine A et al. "Lack of Health Insurance Among Adults Aged 18 to 64 Years: Findings From the 2013 Behavioral Risk Factor Surveillance System." *Preventing chronic disease* vol. 12 E231. 31 Dec. 2015, doi:10.5888/pcd12.150328

193   America's Health Rankings Annual Report." *2019 Annual Report,* United Health Foundation, 2019, assets.americashealthrankings.org/app/uploads/ahr_2019annualreport.pdf

194   *Prison Population By State 2020.* World Population Review, 6 Apr. 2020, worldpopulationreview.com/states/prison-population-by-state

195   Witters, Dan, and Sangeeta Agrawal. *11 Million in U.S. at Serious Risk If Infected With COVID-19.* Gallup, 27 Mar. 2020, news.gallup.com/poll/304643/million-severe-risk-infected-covid.aspx

196 Gates, Bill. *Bill Gates on How to Fight Future Pandemics.* The Economist, 23 Apr. 2020, www.economist.com/by-invitation/2020/04/23/bill-gates-on-how-to-fight-future-pandemics

197 Gates, Bill. *Bill Gates on How to Fight Future Pandemics.* The Economist, 23 Apr. 2020, www.economist.com/by-invitation/2020/04/23/bill-gates-on-how-to-fight-future-pandemics

198 Health Effects Institute. 2018. State of Global Air 2018. Special Report. Boston, MA:Health Effects Institute

199 Brugge, Doug, et al. "Near-Highway Pollutants in Motor Vehicle Exhaust: A Review of Epidemiologic Evidence of Cardiac and Pulmonary Health Risks." *Environmental Health*, vol. 6, no. 1, 2007, doi:10.1186/1476-069x-6-23

200 Schraufnagel, Dean E., et al. "Air Pollution and Noncommunicable Diseases." *Chest*, vol. 155, no. 2, Feb. 2019, pp. 417–426., doi:10.1016/j.chest.2018.10.041

201 Chen, Kai, et al. "Air Pollution Reduction and Mortality Benefit during the COVID-19 Outbreak in China." *The Lancet Planetary Health*, 13 May 2020, doi:10.1016/s2542-5196(20)30107-8

202 Bauwens, M., et al. "Impact of Coronavirus Outbreak on NO 2 Pollution Assessed Using TROPOMI and OMI Observations." *Geophysical Research Letters*, vol. 47, no. 11, 2020, doi:10.1029/2020gl087978

203 *WFP Chief Warns of Hunger Pandemic as COVID-19 Spreads (Statement to UN Security Council).* World Food Programme, 21 Apr. 2020, www.wfp.org/news/wfp-chief-warns-hunger-pandemic-covid-19-spreads-statement-un-security-council

204 Scher, Isaac. *COVID-19 Will Double Number of People Facing Food Crises Unless Swift Action Is Taken.* Business Insider, 21 Apr. 2020, www.wfp.org/news/covid-19-will-double-number-people-facing-food-crises-unless-swift-action-taken

205 Anthem, Paul. *Risk of Hunger Pandemic as COVID-19 Set to Almost Double Acute Hunger by End of 2020.* World Food Programme Insight, 16 Apr. 2020, insight.wfp.org/covid-19-will-almost-double-people-in-acute-hunger-by-end-of-2020-59df-0c4a8072

206 *Hungry South Africans Clash with Police amid Covid-19 Lockdown.* New Straits Times, 14 Apr. 2020, www.nst.com.my/world/world/2020/04/584442/hungry-south-africans-clash-police-amid-covid-19-lockdown

207 Lobo, Andrea. *Hunger Increased by Quarantines Leads to Protests across Latin America.* World Socialist Web Site, 31 Mar. 2020, www.wsws.org/en/articles/2020/03/31/hung-m31.html

208 Abi-habib, Maria, and Sameer Yasir. *India's Coronavirus Lockdown Leaves Vast Numbers Stranded and Hungry.* The New York Times, 29 Mar. 2020, www.nytimes.com/2020/03/29/world/asia/coronavirus-india-migrants.html

209 Fensom, Anthony. *Up In Smoke: Australia's Bushfires Darken Economic Outlook.* For The Diplomat, 13 Jan. 2020, thediplomat.com/2020/01/up-in-smoke-australias-bushfires-darken-economic-outlook

210 Resnick, Brian, et al. *8 Things Everyone Should Know about Australia's Wildfire Disaster.* Vox, 22 Jan. 2020, www.vox.com/science-and-health/2020/1/8/21055228/australia-fires-map-animals-koalas-wildlife-smoke-donate

211 "Monsoon Flooding in Bangladesh." *ShelterBox*, www.shelterbox.org/where-we-work/bangladesh-flooding/.

212 "Cyclone Idai and Kenneth Cause Devastation and Suffering in Mozambique." *UNICEF*, www.unicef.org/mozambique/en/cyclone-idai-and-kenneth

213 *Opinion Survey on COVID-19 and Wildlife Trade in Five Asian Markets.* WWF, 2020, *Opinion Survey on COVID-19 and Wildlife Trade in Five Asian Markets,* c402277.ssl.cf1.rackcdn.com/publications/1328/files/original/WWF_CMS-SINGLES_PAGE.pdf?1585859449

214 Jones, Kate E., et al. "Global Trends in Emerging Infectious Diseases." *Nature*, vol. 451, no. 7181, 21 Feb. 2008, pp. 990–993., doi:10.1038/nature06536

215 Benatar, David. "The Chickens Come Home to Roost." *American Journal of Public Health*, vol. 97, no. 9, Sept. 2007, pp. 1545–1546., doi:10.2105/ajph.2006.090431

216 Benatar, David. "The Chickens Come Home to Roost." *American Journal of Public Health*, vol. 97, no. 9, Sept. 2007, pp. 1545–1546., doi:10.2105/ajph.2006.090431

217 Olival, Kevin J., et al. "Host and Viral Traits Predict Zoonotic Spillover from Mammals." *Nature*, vol. 546, 21 June 2017, pp. 646–650., doi:10.1038/nature22975

218 Zhou, Peng, et al. "Fatal Swine Acute Diarrhoea Syndrome Caused by an HKU2-Related Coronavirus of Bat Origin." *Nature*, vol. 556, 4 Apr. 2018, pp. 255–258., doi:10.1038/s41586-018-0010-9

219 Cui, Jie, et al. "Origin and Evolution of Pathogenic Coronaviruses." *Nature Reviews Microbiology*, vol. 17, 10 Dec. 2018, pp. 181–192., doi:10.1038/s41579-018-0118-9

220 National Research Council (US) Committee on Achieving Sustainable Global Capacity for Surveillance and Response to Emerging Diseases of Zoonotic Origin; Keusch GT, Pappaioanou M, Gonzalez MC, et al., editors. Sustaining Global Surveillance and Response to Emerging Zoonotic Diseases. Washington (DC): National Academies Press (US); 2009. 3, Drivers of Zoonotic Diseases. Available from: https://www.ncbi.nlm.nih.gov/books/NBK215318/

221 Thornton, Philip K. "Livestock Production: Recent Trends, Future Prospects." *Philosophical Transactions of the Royal Society B: Biological Sciences*, vol. 365, no. 1554, 2010, pp. 2853–2867., doi:10.1098/rstb.2010.0134

222 Baldwin, Richard, and Beatrice Weder di Mauro. "Coronavirus monetary policy" *Economics in the Time of Covid-19*, Center for Economic Policy Research, 2020, p. 107

Made in the USA
Monee, IL
16 June 2021

71276379R00090

+MATH FOR MA[RTIANS]

Galaxy Getaway

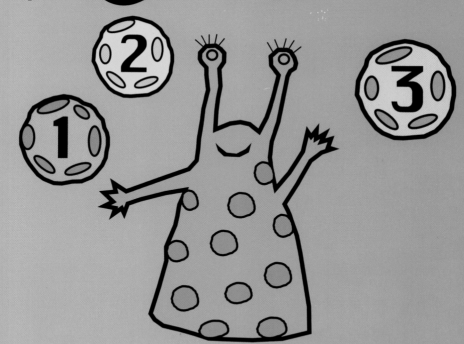

Illustrated by Jane Tassie • Written by Julie Ferris

KINGFISHER

NEW YORK

KINGFISHER
Larousse Kingfisher Chambers Inc.
95 Madison Avenue
New York, New York 10016

First published in 2000
10 9 8 7 6 5 4 3 2 1

1TR/0100/TWP/FR/170ARM

LIBRARY OF CONGRESS CATALOGING—IN—PUBLICATION DATA
Ferris, Julie.
     Galaxy getaway / by Julie Ferris;
illustrated by Jane Tassie.—1st ed.
          p. cm.— (Math for martians)
     Summary: Readers are asked to
solve a variety of math problems
as they journey with Zeno the
Martian across the galaxy.

     ISBN 0-7534-5276-6 (pb)
     1. Mathematics—Study and
teaching (Elementary) [1.
Mathematics—Problems,
exercises, etc. 2. Mathematical
recreations.] I. Tassie, Jane,
ill. II. Title. III. Series.

QA135.5 F485 2000
513—dc21
                    99-040368

Coordinating editor: Laura Marshall

Printed in Singapore

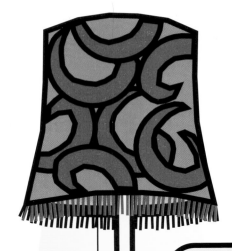

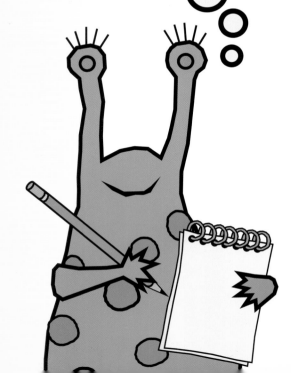

Contents

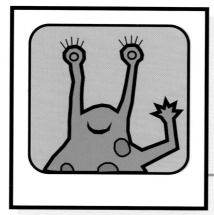

Zeno is only 86 Martian years old (about 10 Earth years). He lives with his mother in Zala, a small city on Mars. Zeno likes adventure, but he is not always very brave.

Zormella is Zeno's cyberpal. She lives in Myria City on planet Numis. She is very practical and always carries a backpack full of useful things.

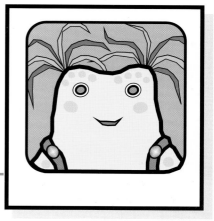

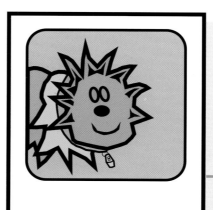

Zarf is a bernum—a small, friendly creature from planet Zib. Bernums are very popular pets throughout the universe.

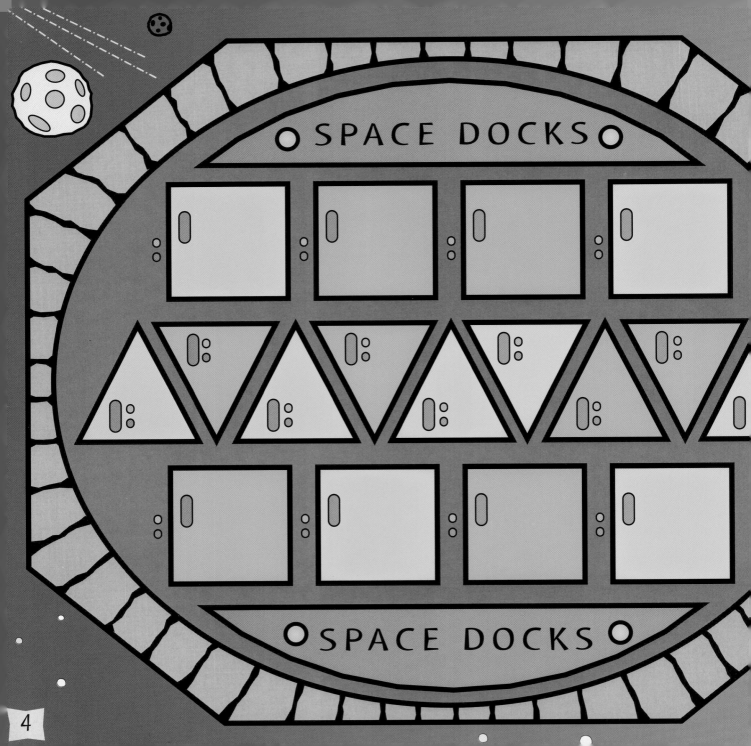

Testing times

Zeno the Martian is very nervous. Today he is taking his space license test. He has flown through a meteor shower and orbited a planet. Now is the hardest part—he has to land his spaceship in a docking port. Can you help him?

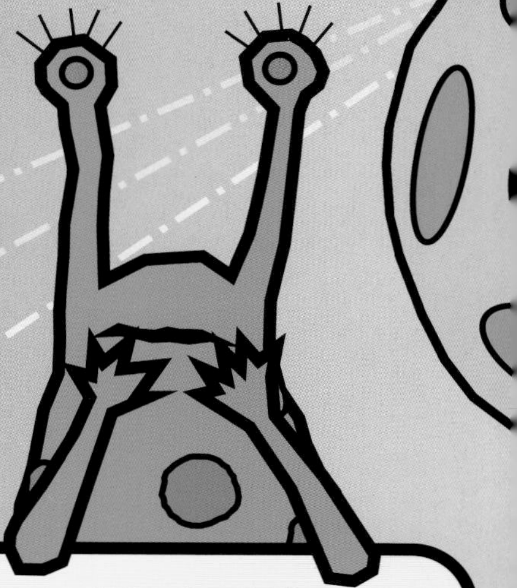

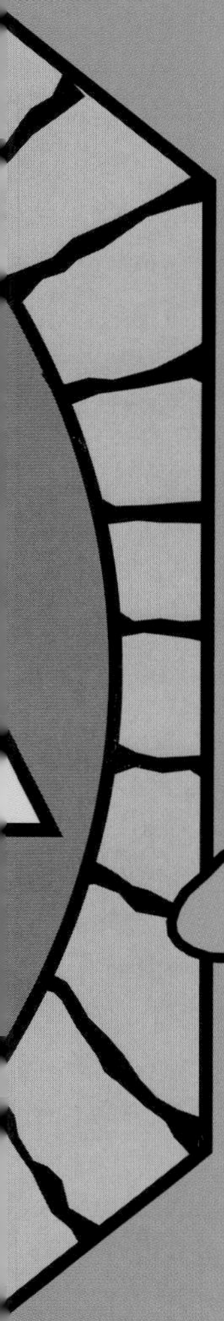

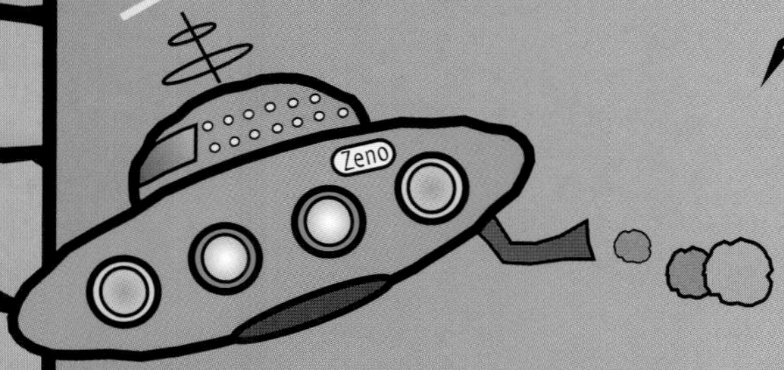

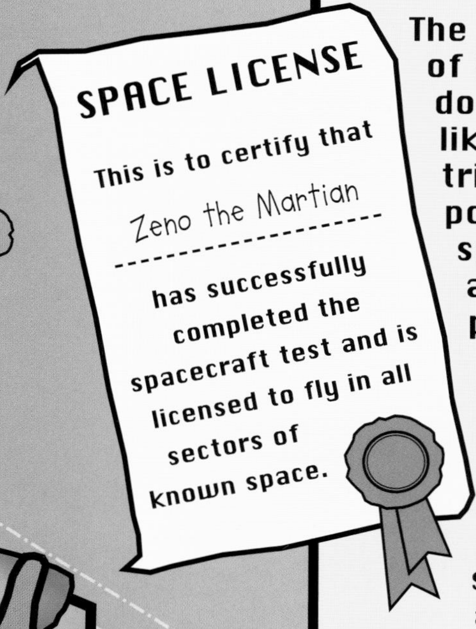

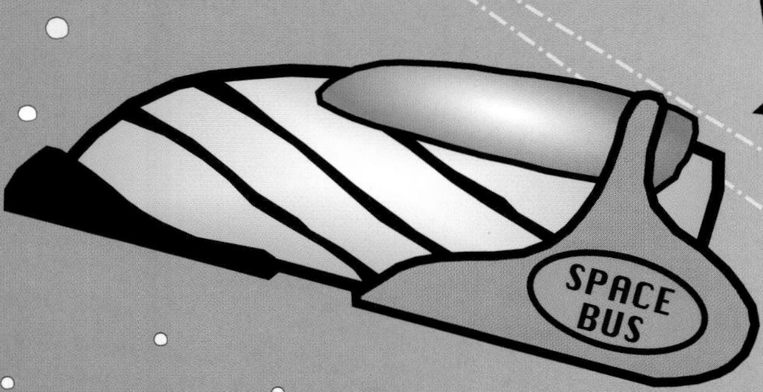

SPACE TEST

The entry pods of Martian space docks are shaped like squares and triangles. Square pods are for space buses, and triangular pods are for smaller spaceships. Empty space pods have yellow doors. How many space bus pods are empty? Zeno is flying a small spaceship. How many pods can he use?

SPACE LICENSE

This is to certify that

Zeno the Martian

----

has successfully completed the spacecraft test and is licensed to fly in all sectors of known space.

SPACE BUS

On board

To celebrate getting his space license, Zeno is taking a special trip. For many Martian years, Zeno has sent intergalactic messages to a cyberpal (a little like a space penpal) in a nearby galaxy. His cyberpal, Zormella, has invited Zeno to visit. It is a long journey, and Zeno needs to make sure his spaceship is shipshape and ready to fly.

Zeno's room

There is a secret safe in the bedroom wall for storing important papers and valuables. To find it, look on the wallpaper for a star that looks different. Starting in the top left corner, count across the rows from left to right. What number star is it?

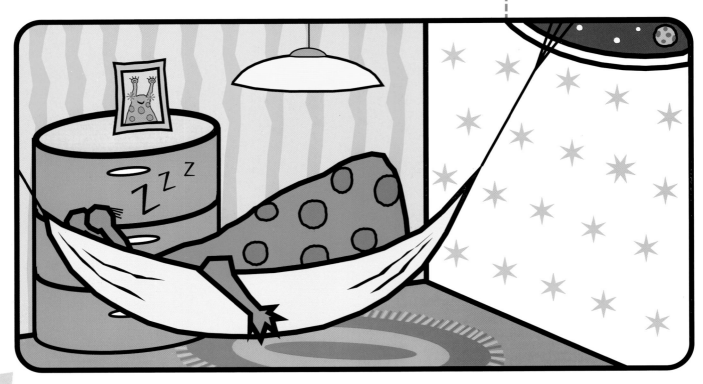

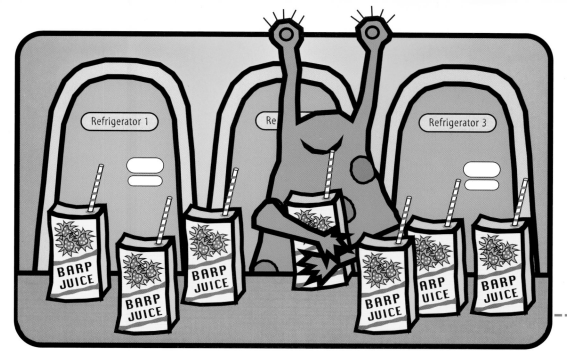

Kitchen

Zeno's favorite drink is barp juice. He usually drinks one carton of barp juice every two hours. The journey will take 12 hours. Does he have enough barp juice?

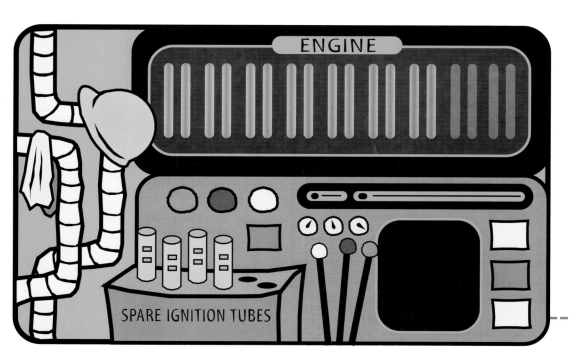

ENGINE

SPARE IGNITION TUBES

Engine room

The spaceship needs eight ignition tubes to take off. Each ignition tube lights up two bars on the engine's display panel. Are there enough ignition tubes loaded?

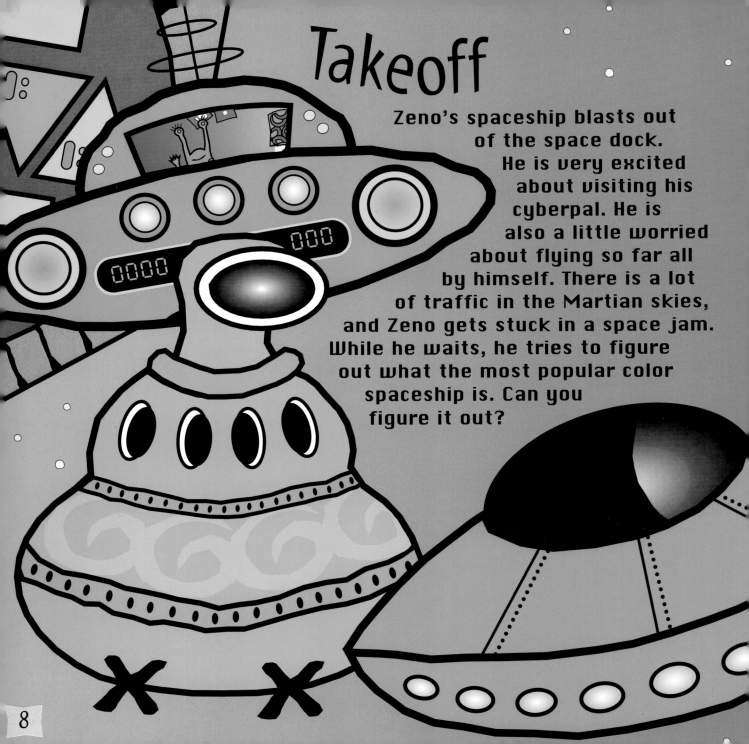

Takeoff

Zeno's spaceship blasts out of the space dock. He is very excited about visiting his cyberpal. He is also a little worried about flying so far all by himself. There is a lot of traffic in the Martian skies, and Zeno gets stuck in a space jam. While he waits, he tries to figure out what the most popular color spaceship is. Can you figure it out?

8

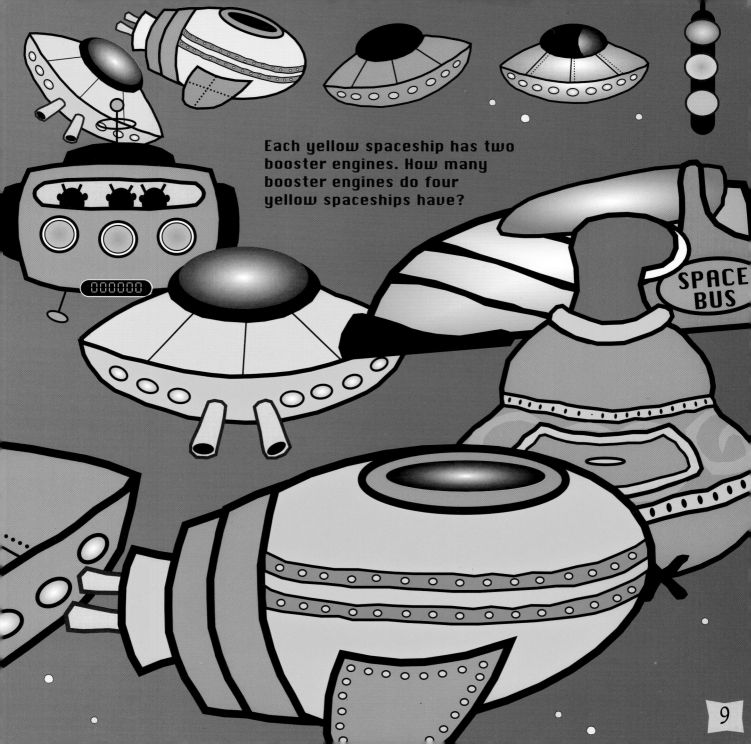

Each yellow spaceship has two booster engines. How many booster engines do four yellow spaceships have?

9

Gas stops

Zeno's spaceship is a real gas-guzzler. He has to stop for gas often or he will get stuck in outer space. Only planets that are part of the five times table have gas supplies.
Can you guide Zeno's spaceship across the galaxy?

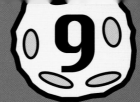
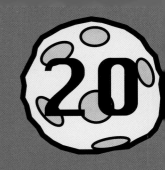
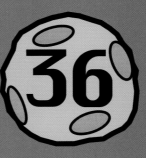
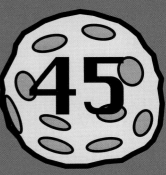
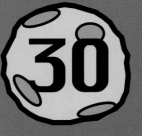
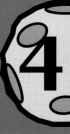
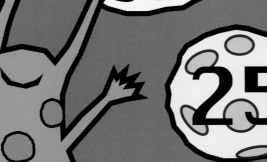
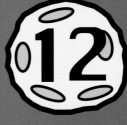
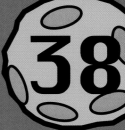
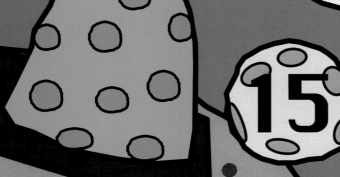
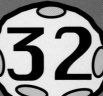
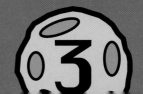

9
20
36
45
3
30
4
25
12
38
15
32
3

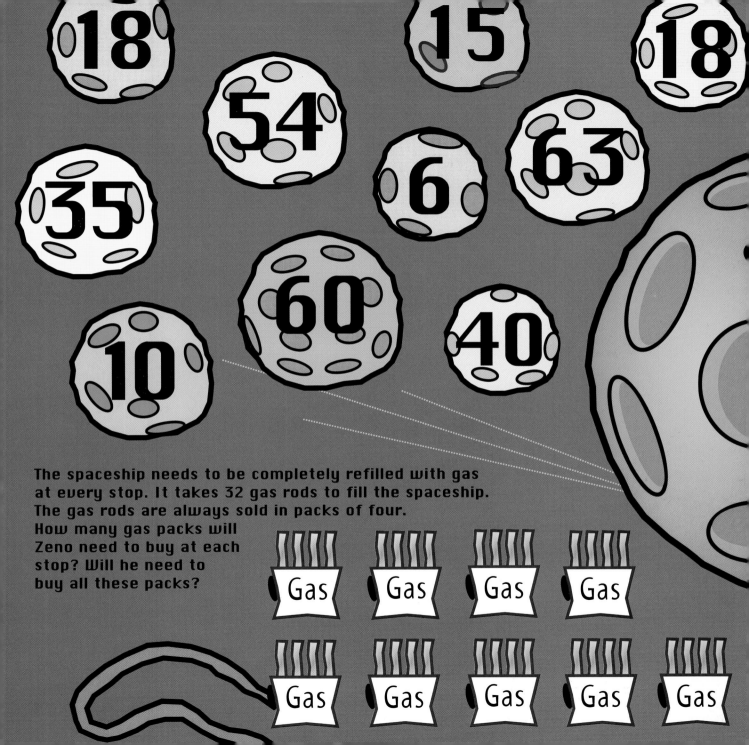

The spaceship needs to be completely refilled with gas at every stop. It takes 32 gas rods to fill the spaceship. The gas rods are always sold in packs of four. How many gas packs will Zeno need to buy at each stop? Will he need to buy all these packs?

Bubble attack

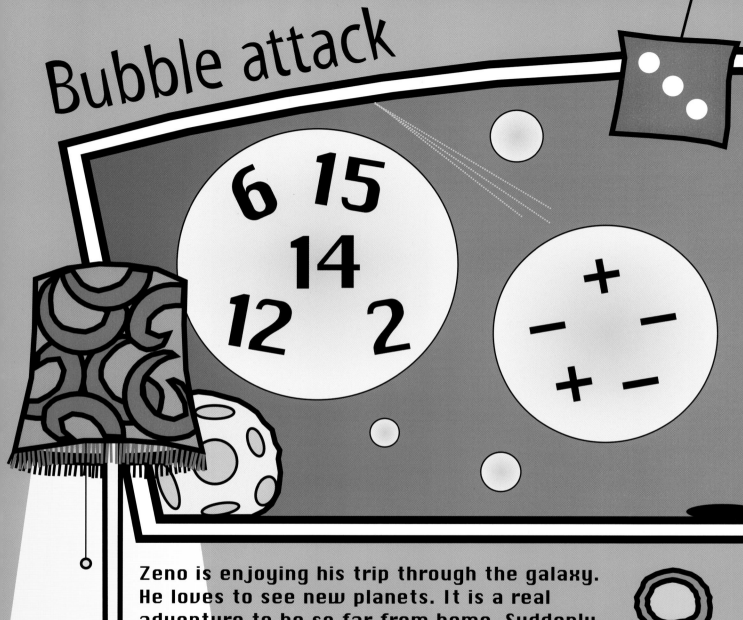

6 15
14
12 2

+
− −
+ −

Zeno is enjoying his trip through the galaxy. He loves to see new planets. It is a real adventure to be so far from home. Suddenly, he sees four space bubbles racing toward his spaceship. He has just a few minutes to burst them before he crashes into them!

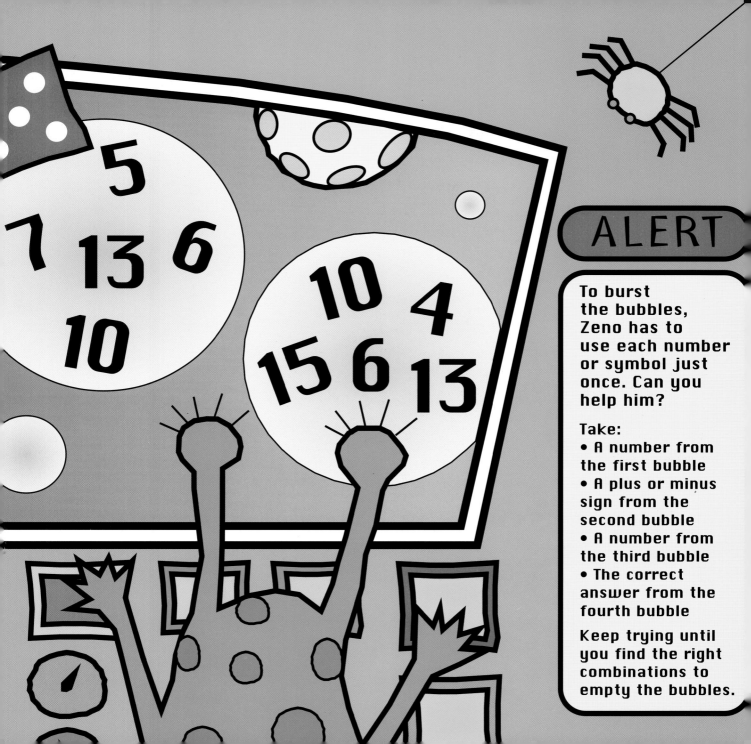

To burst the bubbles, Zeno has to use each number or symbol just once. Can you help him?

Take:
• A number from the first bubble
• A plus or minus sign from the second bubble
• A number from the third bubble
• The correct answer from the fourth bubble

Keep trying until you find the right combinations to empty the bubbles.

Lunchtime!

Bursting bubbles really works up an appetite! Zeno's favorite food is broiled zibbers with mashed space prunes. He is out of zibbers, so he has to land on planet Zib to get some. His turbo food sucker has already collected three zibbers. How many more does he need to make his mom's recipe?

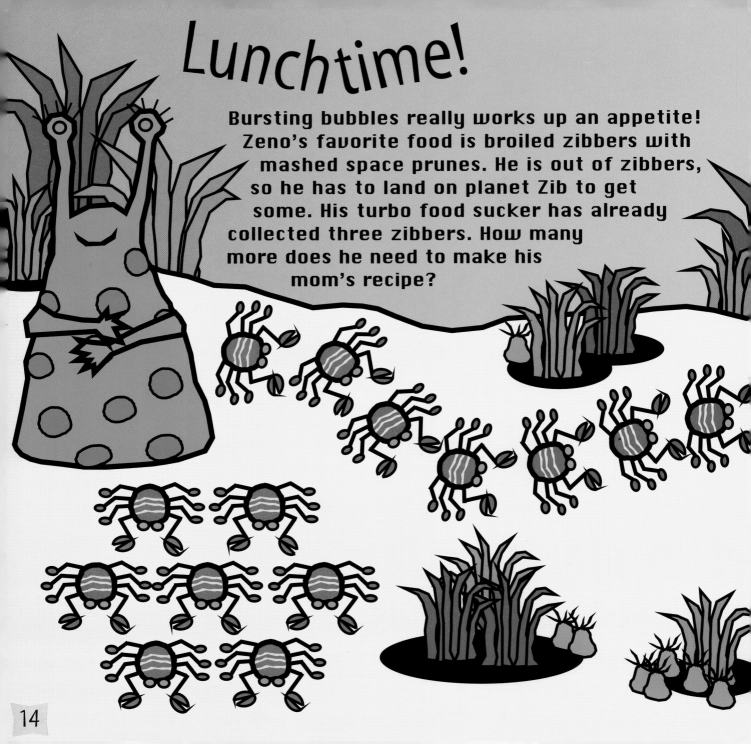

Zibbers are always found in small groups. How many are in each group? How many zibbers are there in total? Can you find enough space prunes for the recipe?

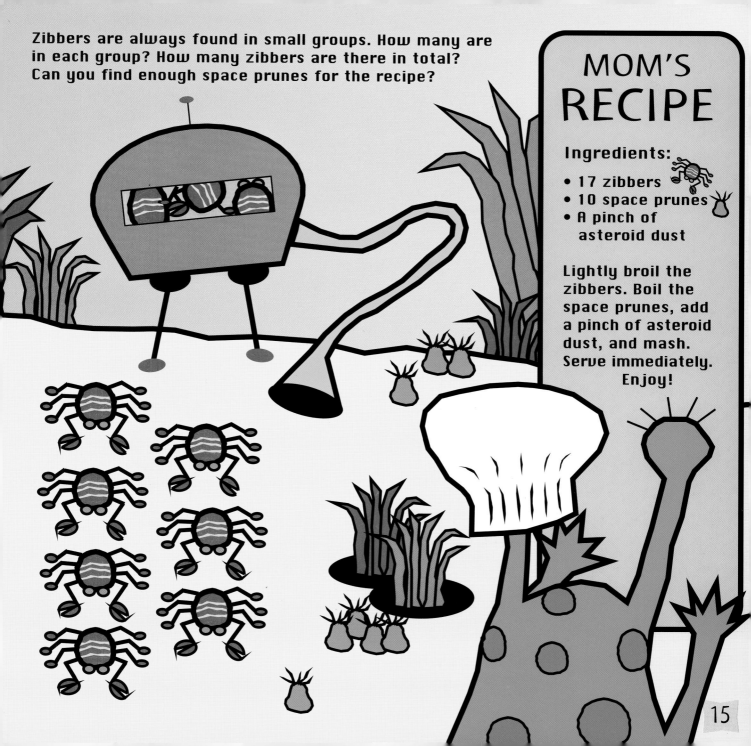

MOM'S RECIPE

Ingredients:

- 17 zibbers
- 10 space prunes
- A pinch of asteroid dust

Lightly broil the zibbers. Boil the space prunes, add a pinch of asteroid dust, and mash. Serve immediately. Enjoy!

Stowaway

As Zeno is eating lunch, he hears a strange rustling noise coming from behind the dresser. Zeno is not the bravest creature in the universe, and at first he is too scared to investigate. Finally he works up the courage to look. He peers into the darkness. Something is creeping toward him....

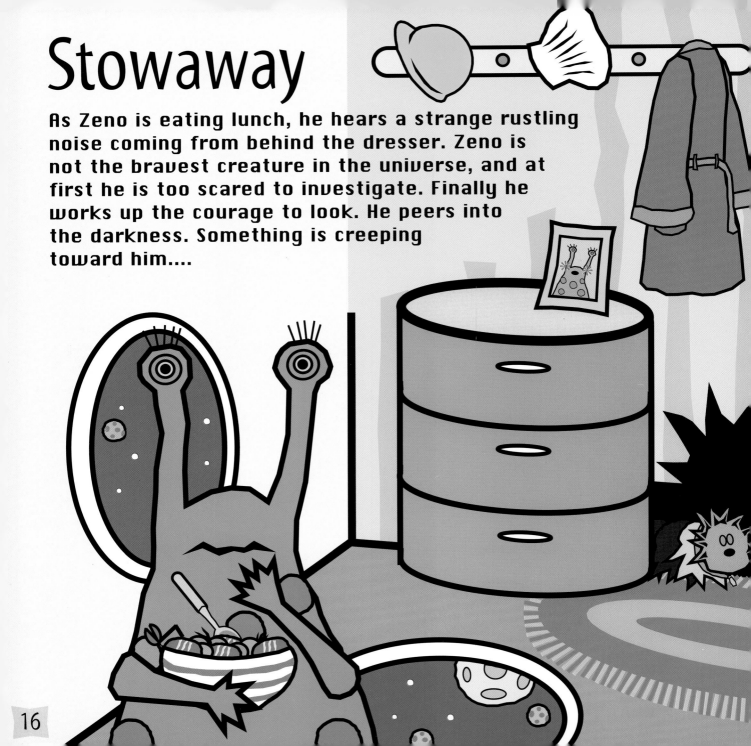

It takes him a few seconds to recognize the strange-looking creature. Then Zeno sees it is just a harmless bernum from the planet Zib. He must have crept on board while Zeno was collecting zibbers.

Hanging around the bernum's neck is a collar with a small message barrel attached to it. Inside, is a message written in code.

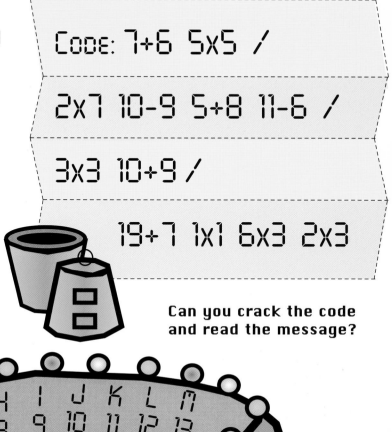

Code: 7+6 5x5 /

2x7 10-9 5+8 11-6 /

3x3 10+9 /

19+7 1x1 6x3 2x3

Can you crack the code and read the message?

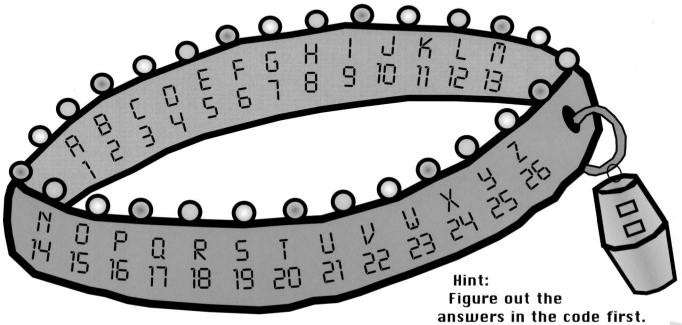

A	B	C	D	E	F	G	H	I	J	K	L	M
1	2	3	4	5	6	7	8	9	10	11	12	13

N	O	P	Q	R	S	T	U	V	W	X	Y	Z
14	15	16	17	18	19	20	21	22	23	24	25	26

Hint:
Figure out the answers in the code first.

Planet Numis

The bernum is friendly. Zeno has always wanted a pet alien, so he takes Zarf the bernum along on his journey. Soon Zeno can see planet Numis. He can't wait to meet his cyberpal, Zormella. Before he lands, Zeno wants to find out more about planet Numis. Here is what he finds on his spaceship's computer.

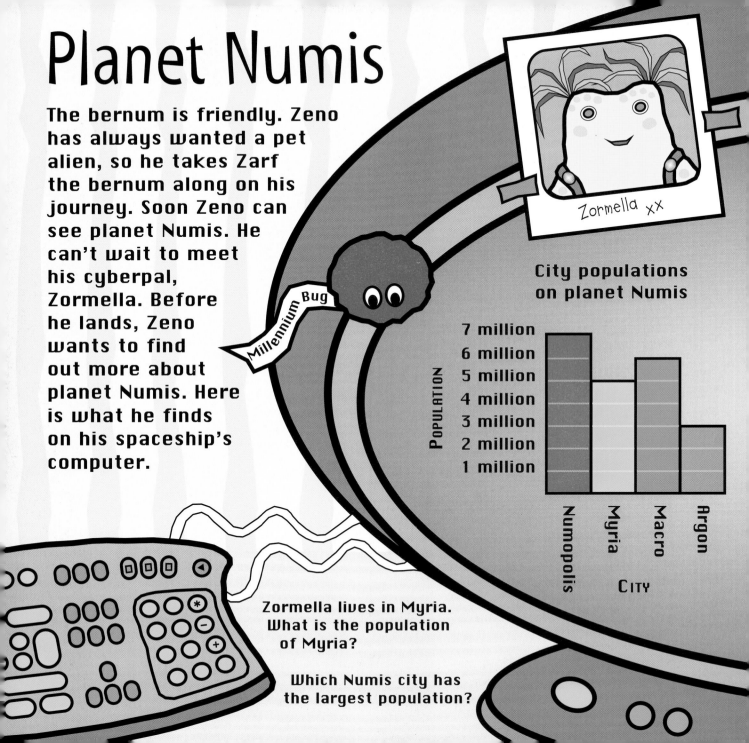

Zormella xx

Millennium Bug

City populations on planet Numis

POPULATION: 7 million, 6 million, 5 million, 4 million, 3 million, 2 million, 1 million

CITY: Numopolis, Myria, Macro, Argon

Zormella lives in Myria. What is the population of Myria?

Which Numis city has the largest population?

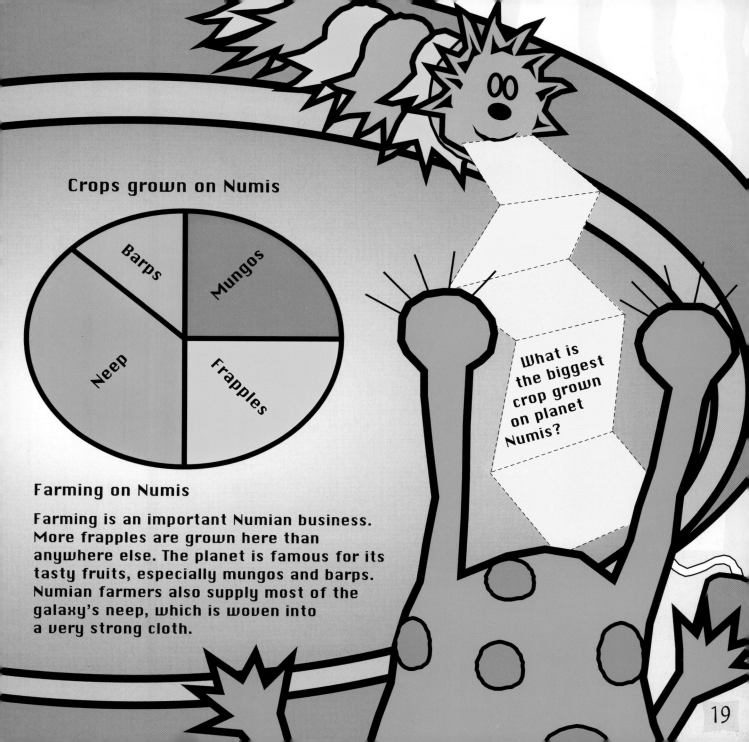

Crops grown on Numis

Barps
Mungos
Neep
Frapples

What is the biggest crop grown on planet Numis?

Farming on Numis

Farming is an important Numian business. More frapples are grown here than anywhere else. The planet is famous for its tasty fruits, especially mungos and barps. Numian farmers also supply most of the galaxy's neep, which is woven into a very strong cloth.

Sightseeing

Zeno lands his spaceship in a Numis docking bay. Zormella is waiting for him. She and Zeno are very happy to finally meet each other. Zeno introduces Zormella to Zarf, and the three of them set off to explore Myria city.

In downtown Myria there is an observation tower with an excellent view. Zeno and Zormella take the turbo-powered elevator to the top of the tower. Zarf doesn't like heights, so he stays behind. How many triangular towers can you see from the top of the observation tower? How many windows are in each triangular tower?

Zeno and Zormella enjoy looking at the view, but where is Zarf? They look all around, but they cannot find him. Can you see where he is?

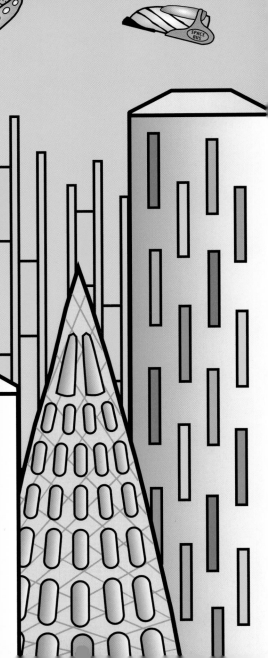

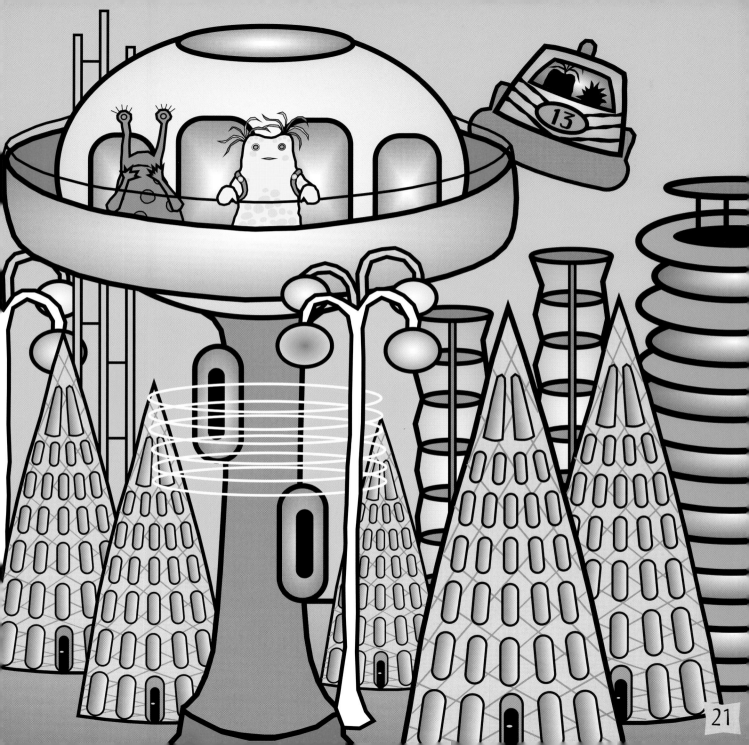

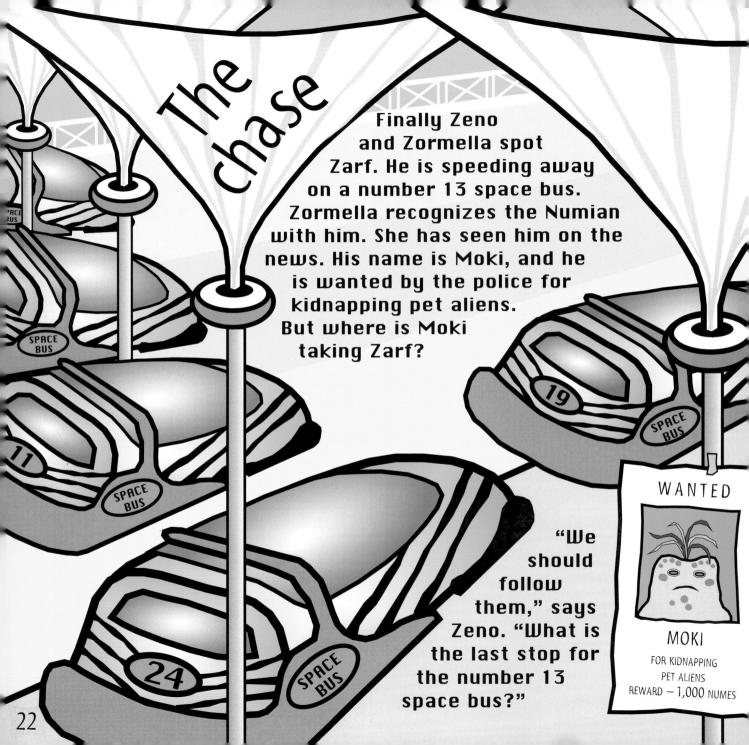

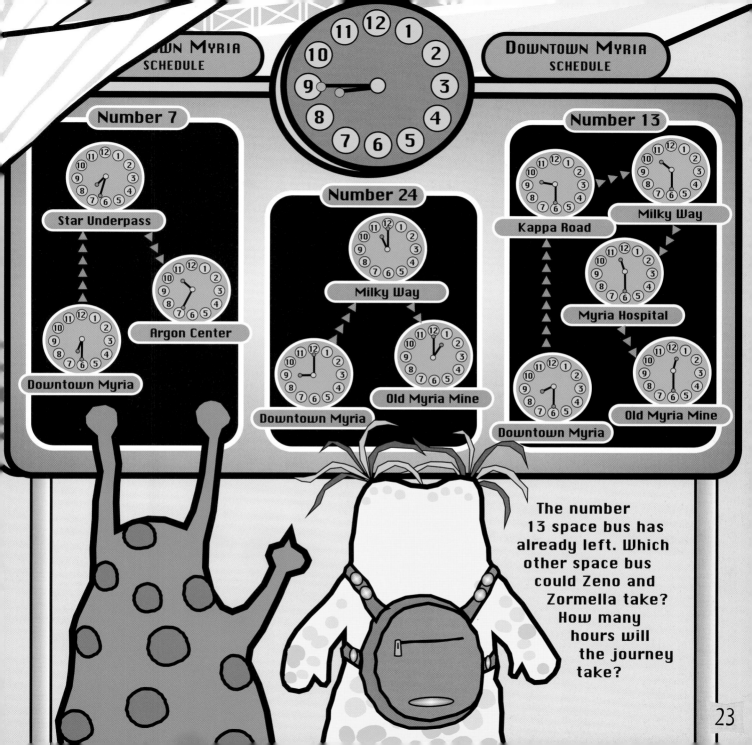

Underground rescue

Zeno and Zormella take the space bus to the Old Myria Mine. At first there is no sign of Zarf or Moki. Then Zormella sees a strange board by the mine entrance. There are four rows of numbers on the board. A number is missing from each row. "If we can figure out the missing numbers, maybe we can unlock the gate," says Zormella. Can you help?

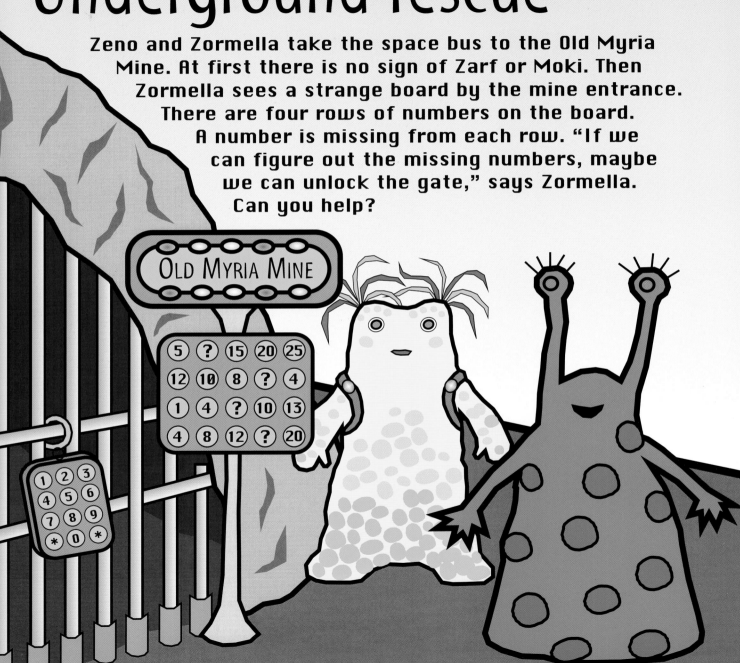

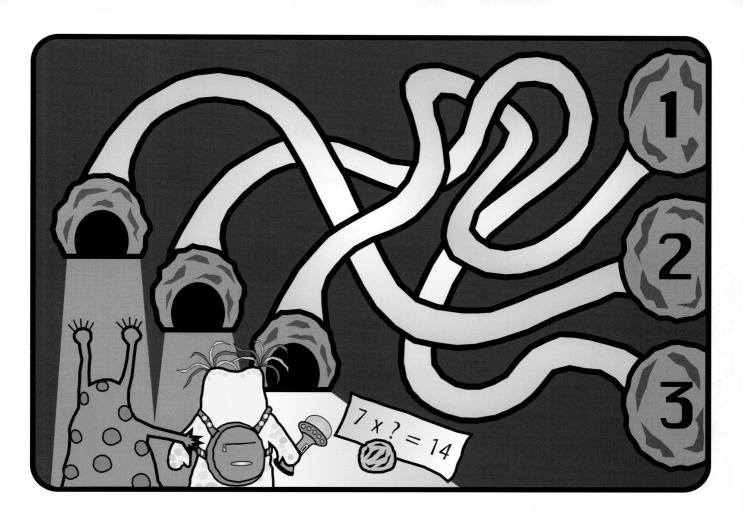

Zeno and Zormella type in the code, and the entrance to the old mine opens. It is very dark inside. Luckily Zormella has a flashlight in her backpack. In front of them are three tunnels. "Which one should we follow?" asks Zormella. Then Zeno sees a scrap of paper on the ground. The paper has numbers on it. Zarf has left them a clue! Can you figure out which tunnel they should go down?

Escape!

The tunnel leads to a large cave. It is packed with cages full of pet aliens. Zarf is in one of the cages. "Moki must be planning to sell the pets in the next galaxy," Zormella whispers. "That's right!" roars Moki. He has spotted the two bold rescuers. "And you can't stop me!"

Zeno has noticed an empty cage hanging right above Moki. He can trap Moki if he can figure out which lever operates the cage. All he has to do is figure out the missing number in the sequence on the cage. Can you help him?

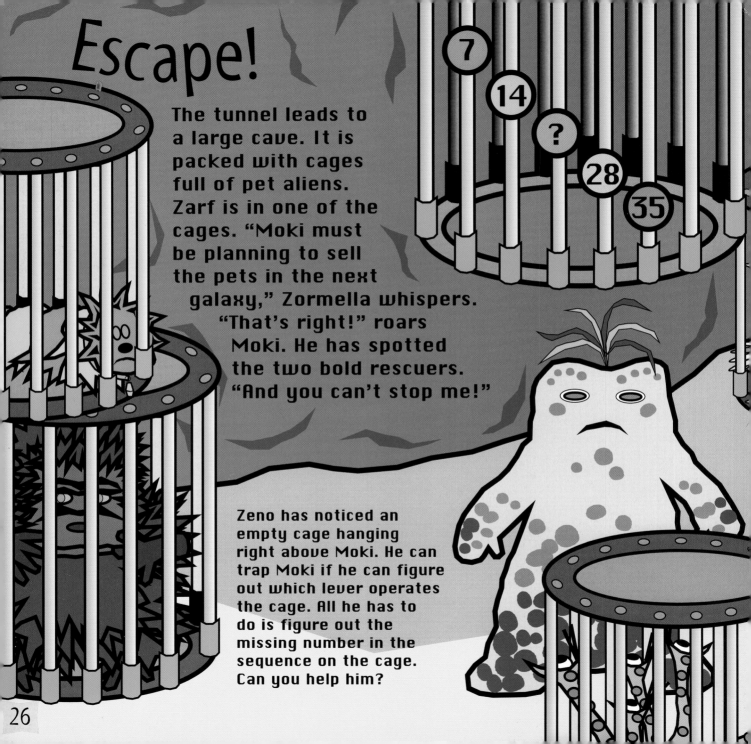

7
14
?
28
35

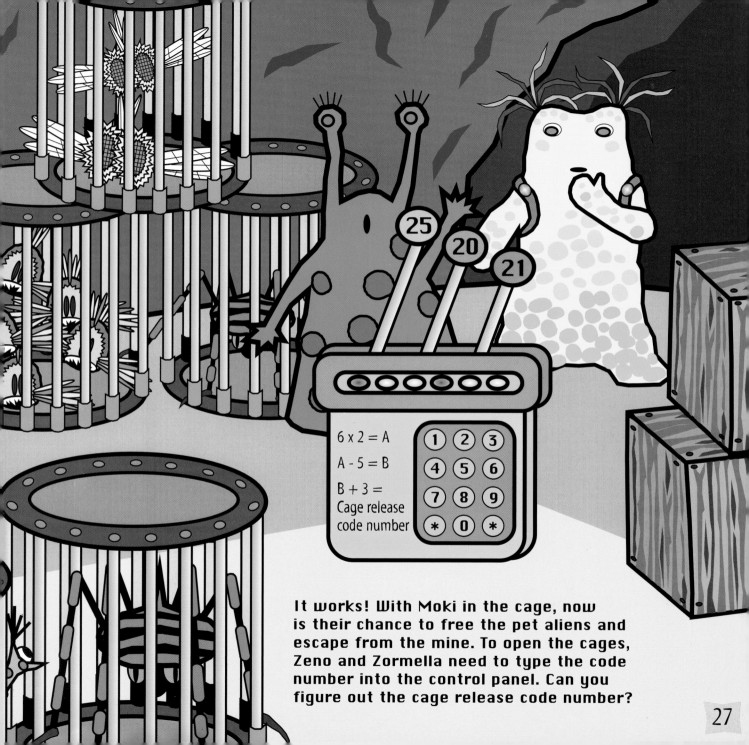

$6 \times 2 = A$

$A - 5 = B$

$B + 3 =$
Cage release
code number

It works! With Moki in the cage, now is their chance to free the pet aliens and escape from the mine. To open the cages, Zeno and Zormella need to type the code number into the control panel. Can you figure out the cage release code number?

Dinnertime!

Zeno, Zormella, and Zarf are very happy to be together again. They all take a space bus to Zormella's house. Their exciting day has made them hungry. Zormella's mother has made a huge meal for them—parberfish sandwiches, zibber potpie, and mungo Jell-O.
"Jumping Jupiter," says Zeno.
"This is delicious!"

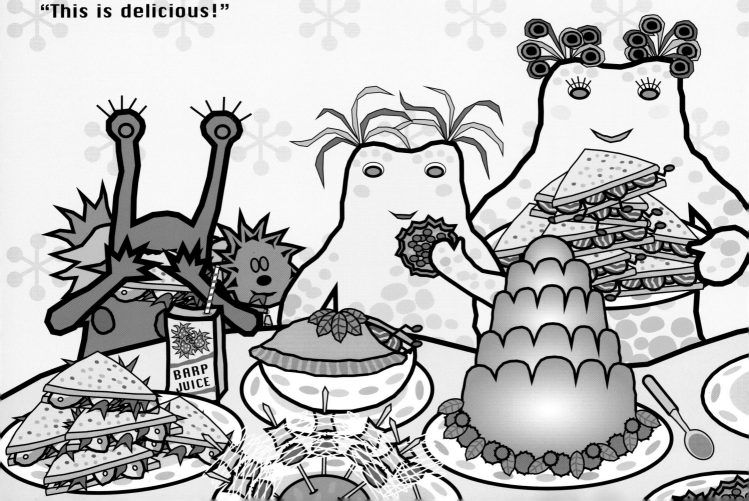

Answers

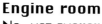

4–5 Testing times

THERE ARE 4 EMPTY SPACE BUS PODS.

Space buses can only park in square pods. Only pods with yellow doors are empty. There are 4 pods that are square and have yellow doors.

ZENO CAN DOCK HIS SMALL SPACESHIP IN 5 PODS.

Small spaceships can only dock in triangle-shaped pods. (Don't forget, an upside-down triangle is still a triangle!) Only pods with yellow doors are empty. There are 5 triangular pods with yellow doors.

6–7 On board

Zeno's room

IT IS STAR NUMBER 9.

Star number 9 has 8 points. All the other stars have 6 points.

Kitchen

YES, ZENO HAS ENOUGH BARP JUICE.

The journey takes 12 hours. Zeno drinks one carton every two hours. There are 6 two-hour blocks in 12 hours ($6 \times 2 = 12$ or $2+2+2+2+2+2=12$). Zeno needs 6 cartons, and he has 7.

Engine room

NO, NOT ENOUGH IGNITION TUBES ARE LOADED.

The spaceship needs 8 ignition tubes to take off. Each ignition tube lights 2 bars, so 16 bars would be lit if enough ignition tubes were loaded ($8 \times 2 = 16$ or $2+2+2+2+2+2+2+2=16$). But only 14 bars are lit. Zeno will have to use one of the spare ignition tubes.

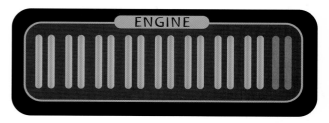

8–9 Takeoff

THE MOST POPULAR COLOR IS ORANGE.

4 YELLOW SPACESHIPS HAVE 8 BOOSTER ENGINES.

Each spaceship has 2 booster engines, so there are 8 engines in all ($4 \times 2 = 8$ or $2+2+2+2=8$).

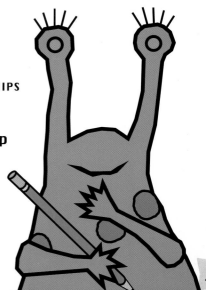

29

10–11 Gas stops

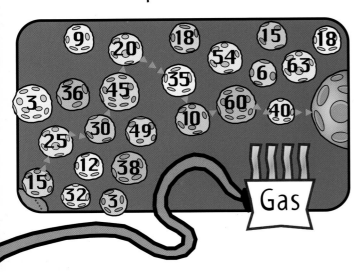

ZENO NEEDS TO BUY **8** GAS PACKS.
Gas rods are sold in packs of 4. Zeno needs 32 gas rods. There are 8 fours in 32 ($8 \times 4 = 32$ or $4+4+4+4+4+4+4+4=32$).
NO, HE WON'T NEED TO BUY ALL THE GAS PACKS IN THE PICTURE.
There are 9 gas packs in the picture, and Zeno only needs 8.

12–13 Bubble attack

$2+13=15$
$6+7=13$
$15-5=10$
$12-6=6$
$14-10=4$

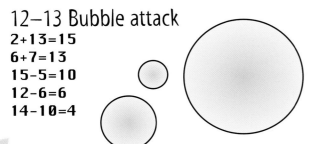

Hint **Try looking at the numbers in the fourth bubble first, and solve them one at a time.**

14–15 Lunchtime!

ZENO NEEDS **14** MORE ZIBBERS.
The recipe calls for 17, and he already has 3 ($17-3=14$).
THERE ARE **7** ZIBBERS IN EACH GROUP. THERE ARE **24** ZIBBERS IN TOTAL.
There are 3 groups of 7 zibbers ($3 \times 7 = 21$ or $7+7+7=21$), plus the 3 zibbers already collected ($21+3=24$).
THERE ARE ENOUGH SPACE PRUNES FOR THE RECIPE.
The recipe needs 10 space prunes, and there are 16 in the picture.

16–17 Stowaway

THE MESSAGE READS: MY NAME IS ZARF.

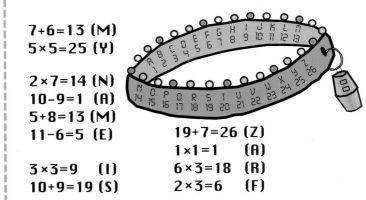

$7+6=13$ **(M)**
$5 \times 5 = 25$ **(Y)**

$2 \times 7 = 14$ **(N)**
$10-9=1$ **(A)**
$5+8=13$ **(M)**
$11-6=5$ **(E)**

$3 \times 3 = 9$ **(I)**
$10+9=19$ **(S)**

$19+7=26$ **(Z)**
$1 \times 1 = 1$ **(A)**
$6 \times 3 = 18$ **(R)**
$2 \times 3 = 6$ **(F)**

18–19 Planet Numis

THE POPULATION OF MYRIA IS **5** MILLION.
Find the top of the bar marked "Myria." Follow the line to the left to see what number is written next to it. This number is the population.
NUMOPOLIS HAS THE LARGEST POPULATION.
7 million NUMIANS LIVE THERE.
The bar for Numopolis is taller than any of the other bars on the bar chart.
NEEP IS THE BIGGEST CROP ON NUMIS.
The section marked "Neep" is the largest on the pie chart.

20–21 Sightseeing

THERE ARE **7** TRIANGULAR TOWERS.
THERE ARE **30** WINDOWS IN EACH TRIANGULAR TOWER.

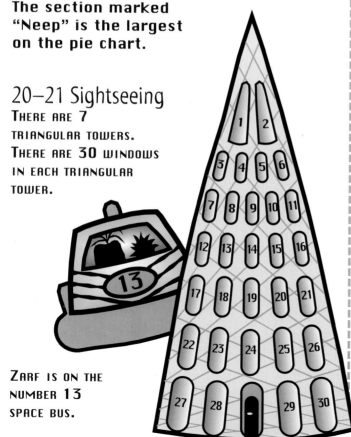

ZARF IS ON THE NUMBER **13** SPACE BUS.

22–23 The chase

THE LAST STOP FOR THE NUMBER **13** SPACE BUS IS THE OLD MYRIA MINE.
ZENO AND ZORMELLA COULD TAKE THE NUMBER **24** SPACE BUS.
It also goes to the Old Myria Mine, and it leaves in 15 minutes!
THE NUMBER **24** SPACE BUS WILL TAKE **4** HOURS TO REACH THE OLD MYRIA MINE.

24–25 Underground rescue

THE MISSING NUMBERS ARE: **10, 6, 7, 16.**

5 **10** 15 20 25
(The numbers go up in fives)
12 10 8 **6** 4 **(Each number is 2 less than the one before it)**
1 4 **7** 10 13 **(Each number is 3 more than the one before it)**
4 8 12 **16** 20 **(The numbers go up in fours)**

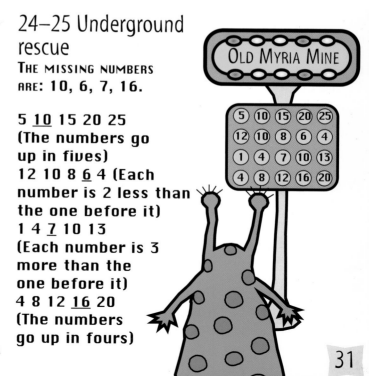

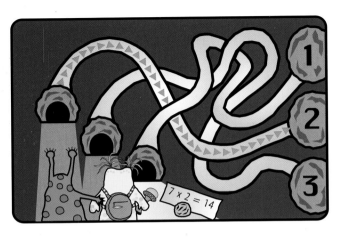

ZENO AND ZORMELLA SHOULD
GO DOWN TUNNEL 2.
$7 \times 2 = 14$ or
$7 + 7 = 14$)

26–27 Escape

ZENO SHOULD PULL
THE LEVER NUMBERED
21.
**The numbers go
up in sevens.**
THE CAGE RELEASE
CODE NUMBER
IS **10.**
$6 \times 2 = \underline{12}$
$\underline{12} - 5 = \underline{7}$
$\underline{7} + 3 = \underline{10}$

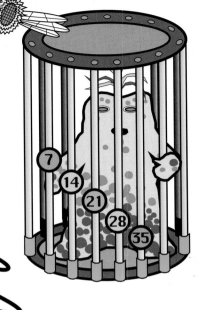

Good-bye!

"It's
time for us
to return to
Mars. I hope
you enjoyed
visiting Zormella
as much as I did. Why
not join us on our next
adventure on Planet Omicron?"

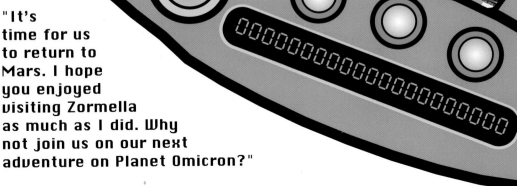